Radionic
Is it for

David V. Tansley DC (USA) honours graduate of
the Los Angeles College of Chiropractic 1965, is
the author of several best-selling books on the
subject of radionics which have revolutionised the
practice of this healing art in modern times. He has
lectured and tutored in parapsychology at the
University of Western Australia and at Murdoch
University, Perth, W.A. For the past decade he
has lectured and held workshops on healing and
the subtle anatomy of man throughout England,
Europe, Australia, South Africa and the United
States. He is considered to be one of the leading
authorities in the field of radionics and the esoteric
constitution of man.

Radionic Healing
Is it for you?

David V. Tansley

with a foreword by
Ian C. B. Pearce
BA, BM, BCh, MRCS, LRCP

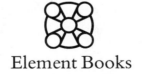

Element Books

Printed and bound in Great Britain by
Billings, Hylton Road, Worcester

Text designed by Humphrey Stone

Cover design by Max Fairbrother

Cover illustration by Ariane Dixon

This book is dedicated to the memory of
MALCOLM RAE
whose unique contribution to radionics
continues to serve practitioners
and patients alike

Contents

Illustrations

Foreword

"The great error of our day," wrote Plato, "in the treatment of the human body, is that physicians first separate the soul from the body." No one could make that accusation against Dr. David Tansley. His view of the true nature of man as being a complex amalgam of the energies of the physical, emotional, intellectual and spiritual levels, intimately associated with, and, indeed, one with the total sum of the cosmic energies, comes through loud and clear. Modern views, just beginning to be assimilated by the medical profession — that the search for the cause of disease must extend beyond the purely physical into the realisation that each individual exists not in a state of isolation, but is swimming in an immense sea of cosmic energy, of which he or she is an integral part, and in so being, is a part of all his or her fellow creatures — are here enunciated with devastating precision and clarity. Dr. Tansley has brought the whole concept of disease away from idiopathic malfunction of cells and organs into a spiritual dimension, and fused together the intuitive perceptions of eastern thought with western analysis and logic. Disease is here viewed not as the consequence of external attack, but as self-created, out of patterns of thought and emotional attitudes; and the healing of that disease as being the sequel to the correction and rebalancing of the energy systems of which the individual is composed. Radionics is seen as being a practical way of assisting the all important process of rebalancing these energy systems.

This is not a book which will commend itself to orthodoxly trained physicians. It will be seen by them as a powerful attack on their traditional position as the guardians of the health of the public, and on the authority which they wield over the lives of their patients. Although science has now been forced to accept the existence of the electro-magnetic field in association with living bodies, and even that this field can be affected by other fields in the universe, the concept that emotions, thoughts and even the spirit, can exist in their own right, and can influence the behaviour of physical bodies, is not one which readily commends itself to those who still believe that thought is the product of brain cell activity. Once the practices outlined in this book become more generally applied in the healing field, the traditional approach of the medical profession will become progressively eroded, and the role of the orthodox physician superfluous.

To most people the term 'radionics' is evocative of the micro-chip and the world of the computer — something which is past their comprehension, unless they have been specially trained in this field. The idea that it is actually possible for someone sitting in England to arrive at an accurate understanding of not only a disease process, but also of the total personality, of a patient acrosss the other side of the world in, say, Australia is so improbable as to seem totally beyond belief. However, the scientists of a generation ago held the same views about telepathy, only to have it conclusively demonstrated by Ravitz that the phenomenon was a fact. In a similar way many scientists today, despite the existence of many well documented examples, refuse to accept that precognition can occur. Time and space, it seems, are dimensions of the material world, which is only one part of the cosmic whole. Those who read Dr. Tansley's book will have a better understanding of these facts.

The phenomena of intuitive perception and of distance healing are nothing new. They have been with us since the beginning of time and many examples are to be found in the pages of the Bible. Many healers and prayer groups today operate in this way. Dowsing for water and for minerals has been an accepted practice for generations. The toxic effects of many chemicals and minerals are today becoming widely recognised, and are, indeed, giving rise to the development of a new branch of medicine, that of medical ecology. The ideas of Hahnemann that 'like heals like' have been around for over a century, while the Bach flower remedies are widely used by a great number of people. Dr. Tansley weaves all these apparently disconnected fragments into a coherent tapestry of understanding, which will greatly strengthen the ideas of those who believe that medicine is currently on a downward and self-destructive path.

The term 'holistic medicine' is freely bandied around at the present time, and to most people it appears to be synonymous with 'alternative'. In fact, this is totally inaccurate. Holistic means treatment of the whole, and holistic medicine implies the treatment by physicians of the totality of man — spirit, mind and body — instead of confining treatment, as most doctors do at present, to the physical body only. It implies a recognition by the doctor of man's essentially spiritual nature, and of the homoeostatic — or self-healing — power of the creature. It also implies the recognition by the patient of his or her own responsibility and involvement in both the disease-making and the healing process. In this respect radionics is truly holistic in the fullest sense of the word. The radionic analysis and interpretation to the patient, whatever his level of understanding, can only help in this self-healing process. My only reservation rests in the continuing use of the word 'treatment', which seems to convey to the patient that something is being done *to* him or her by an external agency, instead of conveying the idea of assistance in re-balancing the energy systems and reinforcing the power of self-healing.

The final and $64,000 question must inevitably be, 'Does it work?' "Radionics is a load of rubbish," one prominent American surgeon said to the writer. "But," he added with a wry smile, "it works!" Dr. Tansley explains how and why it works. And work it certainly does, as I have good reason to know, since for a number of years I received radionic assistance from a greatly respected and much loved teacher of radionics for a chronic bowel complaint, on one occasion over a distance of 6,000 miles.

Radionics is still ahead of its time. There will be many who read this excellent book who will dismiss it with a contemptuous shrug of the shoulders, and, perhaps, the sneer: "Well, if you believe that, you will believe anything." However, the passage of time and the dedicated work and teaching of such people as Dr. Tansley and his colleagues will ensure its continuation. Eventually it is probable that it will supercede orthodox medicine. My only regret is that by that time I shall be outside the time-space continuum, and shall have to observe it from another dimension.

IAN C. B. PEARCE. BA, BM, BCH, MRCS, LRCP

What is Radionics?

By its very nature radionics is difficult to define. If one searches through the various writings on the subject, it soon becomes evident that a precise definition is lacking for this unique and remarkable healing art. You will not for example find the word 'radionics' in the dictionary. If you were to question a cross-section of the public, asking them, "what is radionics?" the chances are that few, if any, would be able to give the correct answer. Some might hazard a guess that it has something to do with radio, but then they would be completely wrong. Why is it difficult to define radionics, surely if something exists it can be defined? The difficulty arises, I believe, because radionics has such breadth and depth, such potential, and its scope is so universal that it cannot be comfortably confined within the limited framework of the beliefs and concepts that govern our lives in the everyday world. Radionics in all of its aspects breaks through the barriers of orthodox knowledge. It is a healing art that expands our view of human nature; it is vitalistic rather than mechanistic. It broaches the barriers that exist between science, philosophy and religion and above all it is concerned with the whole person. Having said this I must try to create some kind of definition around which the various aspects of radionics can cluster, in order to give you an impression of the whole.

Put simply, radionics is a system of distant diagnosis and treatment, which utilises the human faculties of extra-sensory perception in conjunction with certain specially designed instruments, to determine the underlying root causes of disease in a living organism. It is a healing art that has its roots in twentieth century medicine, but is unique in that its techniques of diagnosis and treatment consciously and deliberately employ the higher faculties of the mind, which science for the most part has seen fit to deny.

Our society in general is conditioned to a rather narrow view of the world, and it is this conditioning which cries out against the concept that it is possible to diagnose what is wrong with someone who lives many miles away, perhaps even on the other side of the world. Our intellect with its rational and logical approach to life says that such an act as distant diagnosis is not logical, therefore it cannot be effectively carried out. The intellect demands that in order to know what is wrong with a patient, the practitioner must see and examine them physically. Many people's thinking stops right at this point because their approach to life is based on what is known as intellectual knowledge, which is fine in so far as it goes. There is however another form of knowledge, and that is intuitive knowledge. We have all experienced this many times in our lives; we often know things without knowing why or how we know them. We have pre-visions, feelings or impressions of things not visible to the physical senses. In fact if we take time to observe how our minds function, it is quite amazing just how often the intuitive faculty demonstrates itself. Most of us have experienced the strong impression or thought of a friend or relative, only to have them phone within the next minute or so. Or a letter might turn up in the mail from a friend you have not had contact with for years, preceeded by thoughts of that person who has not even entered your mind for ages. These are not coincidences, but the higher faculties of the mind in action.

The trouble is that the logical aspects of our mind tend to automatically shut out recognition of these inner mind-to-mind impressions. What happens when you pick up the phone and it is the friend you were just thinking about, a friend you perhaps have not been in touch with for months, perhaps even years? You evince surprise, then say, "I was just thinking of you." Both of you laugh and the incident is submerged and effectively dismissed. There are more important things to discuss than the clear evidence of some subtle and quite remarkable form of communication that took place prior to the phone ringing. Later we will look at this phenomenon in some detail because it will help us to understand in some measure, just how radionic distant diagnosis and treatment work.

Although we are for the most part dominated by our intellectual and logical mind, the remarkable fact is that many of the greatest discoveries made in science have come not so much through the use of the intellectual faculties, although no one would deny their importance, but through intuitive insights, flashes of inspiration borne out of day-dreaming, musing and inner reflection. Not least of these was Einstein's Theory of Relativity, which radically changed man's view of the world.

While the intellect by its very nature works within certain limits, the intuitive faculty of man, when developed, appears to be unlimited in its scope to comprehend and express the mysteries that underlie our physical universe and the world we live in. Clearly to be able to diagnose what is wrong with a person at a distance, and then, having determined the cause of their ill health, to treat it from a distance, is a remarkable phenomenon. But it is one that lies well within the province of a sensitive and properly trained radionic practitioner. We are rapidly entering the era of the mind, and even now as we look at some of its remarkable capacities, it is evident that the human mind is a thing of awesome power with abilities and capacities we have barely begun to tap. These of course, when harnessed and guided by the highest motives, can be used to heal and bring harmony to life in many unusual ways, often in cases where all else has failed.

Today more and more people are discovering radionics through friends, relatives or associates, and turning to this form of healing in an effort to rid themselves of health problems which have not responded to other types of treatment. The beauty of radionic treatment is of course its compatibility with any other form of therapy, and it is frequently used in conjunction with homoeopathic medicines, the biochemic tissue salts and the Bach flower remedies. Above all, radionics is a non-invasive approach to healing, devoid of the unpleasant side effects so often associated with drugs.

Radionics of course is not a panacea, but it has the advantage over other methods in that, through controlled use of the mind the practitioner has access to levels and areas of information in respect of the patient's health which lie well beyond the physical, wherein deeply ingrained disease-causing factors may be harboured. The practitioner may find for example, that the patient has a high level of toxic residue left over from measles. Having had the disease as a child or been innoculated, few of us would give it another thought, but it is a fact that the relatively innocuous childhood diseases may leave highly toxic residues which can in many instances undermine general health to a greater or lesser degree. Through radionics these toxins can be identified and eliminated, thus paving the way to better health. Further on in the book, we will take a look at the effects of toxins in some detail, and outline just how they affect our health adversely. We will consider for example the effect of toxins from aluminium cooking-ware, and those from the silver-mercury amalgam fillings in teeth. These are just two factors that are so commonplace in our lives that we seldom, if ever, give them a thought, and yet if you are sensitive to these substances they could literally devastate your health.

Having briefly defined radionics it is clear that what has been written raises a whole host of other questions. As I said previously, radionics is hard to define, somehow it requires more than that, it demands explanation. If I say, for example, that, broadly speaking, medicine is the use of drugs and surgery to restore health and prevent disease, you will understand what I am saying because your mind is familiar with these principles and requires no further elaboration or explanation. But when I say that radionics is a form of instrumented distant diagnosis and treatment that utilises the human faculties of extra-sensory perception, we are at once outside the realm of everyday beliefs and concepts. The definition as I said, demands an explanation and in so doing immediately raises a host of other questions such as — how does radionics work? How can a practitioner determine what is wrong with a patient without having seen them, and how could they possibly treat them at a distance? What does a radionic diagnosis cover? How is it done and how is treatment given? What diseases can be treated by this method?

I shall endeavour to answer these questions as simply and as clearly as possible, but before doing so it will be necessary to deal with the most fundamental question that radionics raises — what is the nature of man and the world he lives in? In other words is life a strictly physical phenomenon as the behaviourists and mechanists would have us believe, or is there more to life and man than meets the physical senses?

As I mentioned earlier, radionics occupies a position between science and philosophy, in fact between science and religion if you like. It is a healing art that interfaces with many other fields of human endeavour, particularly those mentioned above, and it brings with it the quality of synthesis. This is perhaps one of its most unique and fas-

cinating characteristics because it forces us to seek for a
working hypothesis for radionics by drawing upon material
from scientific, religious and philosophical sources in order
to come to some understanding of the observable phenomena that arise out of the practice of this unusual healing
art. Undoubtedly radionics is a complex subject, but having
said this, its fundamental principles which we shall explore,
are in themselves quite simple. However before dealing
with the modus operandi of radionics I think it best if we
look briefly at its history and some of the individuals who
have contributed to this field.

2

A Brief History of Radionics

The founder of radionics was a Dr. Albert Abrams who was born in 1863. By any standards he was an outstanding individual who devoted his entire life, and the bulk of his inherited fortune to research in the medical field. Abrams was the son of a rich merchant who lived in San Francisco, but rather than follow in his father's footsteps he studied medicine. In fact he completed his studies at such an early age that he was too young to be awarded his degree. Feeling that he could further his studies elsewhere, he learned German and enrolled in one of the finest medical schools of the time at the University of Heidelberg. Completing the entire course of study he graduated with the degrees of M.D. and M.A., plus first class honours and the gold medal of the University. He subsequently did extensive post-graduate work throughout Europe with such men as Virchow, Von Helmholtz, Frerichs and Wassermann, all of whom were to become giants in the medical world of their time.

After returning to California, Abrams became Professor of Pathology and ultimately Director of Clinical Medicine at Leland Stanford University. He was a fellow of the American Medical Association and the author of at least twelve books. Before long he acquired a national reputation as a specialist in diseases of the nervous system. Despite the fact that he was a millionaire and could well have taken life easy, Abrams lived for his work and used his fortune to further medical research.

Had Abrams remained in the mainstream of medicine he would probably have been fêted by his peers; instead he was to make a discovery that would bring attack and vilification upon him from all quarters of the medical and scientific community. His discovery happened quite accidentally during the routine examination of a middle-aged male patient who had a malignant ulcer on his lip. Towards the completion of his examination, Abrams gently percussed the abdomen of the patient to define the border of the stomach. To his surprise instead of a hollow sound, the percussive note was dull and heavy. Abrams was puzzled so he palpated the patient's abdomen to see if any mass was present, but this proved negative. Abrams, unlike most other physicians who would have given little thought to the phenomenon, continued to percuss the patient's abdomen. After several hours he had established that the dull note only sounded when the patient faced west. If he faced in any other direction or lay down the note became normal. Abrams knew that he had made a remarkable discovery, and he followed it up by bringing in a whole series of patients from the clinic who had cancer. Without exception everyone of them exhibited the same area of dullness above the navel. This reaction became known as 'The Electronic Reaction of Abrams', or 'E.R.A.', and it provided the basis for Abrams' theory that disease was not so much a matter of cellular imbalance as an imbalance of the electrons of the atoms of the body. He theorised in fact, that disease was a form of radiating energy which could be detected by E.R.A. methods. This in effect was the beginning of what was to become known as 'radionics'. The word radionics is derived from the words 'radiations' and 'electronics'. *Radi* from radiations, and *onics* from electronics. It is a strange word perhaps, but quite descriptive.

Fired by his discovery, Abrams began carefully to examine a whole series of patients with specific diseases, and he found that areas of dullness could be defined for each condition. Tuberculosis, for example, evoked a dull note from an area just beneath the navel. Streptococcal infection to the left of it, and malaria and pneumococcus well below and to the left and right respectively. Abrams was getting along fine with his mapping of disease identification areas, when he found that the area for syphilis superimposed itelf precisely over that for cancer. This obviously presented a problem because now he had to find a way to distinguish one reaction from another, and clearly there were so many diseases that sooner or later he would run out of space on the human abdomen anyway.

Abrams reasoned that if the disease patterns were a form of electronic radiation it might be possible to measure them with a variable resistance type of apparatus. So he experimented with a variable resistance box, which in today's world of electronic sophistication would be considered crude in the extreme. But it worked, and Abrams found that cancer could be measured at 50 ohms and syphilis would only give a reaction at 55 ohms. So he had a way of measuring disease reactions and distinguishing them one from another. It was a remarkable breakthrough and Abrams compiled an atlas of disease areas and their resistance in ohms which became known as 'rates'. Today all disease conditions and organ systems of the body have 'rates', or numerical values, which are used for diagnostic and treatment purposes in radionic practice. So Abrams had made a fundamental contribution to what was to become radionics.

Constant experimentation led Abrams to develop his instrumentation. He called the resistance box a 'Bio-dynamometer' and to this he added a circular container known as the 'Dynamiser' which held the blood sample of the patient. Abrams no longer percussed the abdomen of each patient but used instead the abdomen of one healthy young man who became known as the 'Subject'. In this manner Abrams could check any number of patients

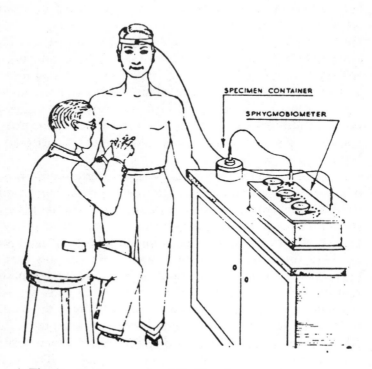

SPECIMEN CONTAINER

SPHYGMOBIOMETER

1. The diagnostic apparatus of Abrams, illustrating the use of the abdomen of a healthy male subject as a detector.

without them having to be present, and the system worked just as effectively as if they had been there.

It does not take much imagination to realise the response Abrams would get from his medical colleagues, they were horrified, and in no time at all he found himself under increasing attack, not only from his colleagues but from the scientific community at large. Despite the attacks mounted against him, Abrams attracted a constant stream of physicians, chiropractors and osteopaths from all over the

United States, Britain and Europe, who were eager to learn his revolutionary new techniques. Not least amongst those who used Abrams' methods was the British physician Sir James Barr who was later to write a book in defence of Abrams' work — he hailed it, in fact, as the medical discovery of the century.

Another instrument was to follow the development of the Biodynamometer which was primarily for diagnostic work, and that was the Oscilloclast which was used for treatment. This instrument was attached to the patient by leads and employed pulsed, weak electro-magnetic energy which was modified by the appropriate treatment rates. The patient would sit for upwards of an hour attached to the Oscilloclast while the energies from the instrument flowed through his body bringing balance to the electrons of the atoms. In this manner practitioners of the E.R.A. methods got spectacular results. It seemed to many that a whole new era in medicine was about to unfold, but they, like Abrams were due to be disappointed. Abrams, driven by his daemon, virtually died on his feet in the laboratories where he had striven so hard to find new ways to relieve the sufferings of his fellow man. In England the pressure had mounted to such a pitch that the medical authorities were forced to form a committee to examine the claims for Abrams' work.

In 1924 an investigating team was set up under the direction of Sir Thomas Horder (later to become Lord Horder), and between June 7th and August 24th a series of twenty-five tests were run in Glasgow. The operator of the instrument, in this instance a Boyd's Emanometer, was to attempt to distinguish phials which contained homoeopathic sulphur in a 10M potency from phials containing a similar amount of neutral material. One by one these phials were introduced into the circuit of the instrument, unseen by the operator. When the tests were completed the investigating committee were staggered to find that the contents of every phial in every test had been correctly identified. At first the committee tried to brush this accuracy off as chance but when the odds were computed at 1 to 33,554,432 against this happening, they had reluctantly to concede that the claims for Abrams' instrument and the effectiveness of the technique were valid.

Despite the fact that this rigid testing by a select team of physicians and physicists had shown that the Electronic Reaction of Abrams worked with a high degree of accuracy, medicine as a body, turned its collective back on this discovery and ignored it in the hope that it would go away. Fortunately it did not, and more and more practitioners employed the method. New pioneers emerged to extend the work by designing more sophisticated instruments and outlining more effective diagnostic and treatment techniques.

These pioneers were legion and for the most part the records of their research work are lost or lie hidden in dusty attics or cellars throughout America. The 1930's saw the emergence of Dr. Ruth Drown, a chiropractor practising in Hollywood, California. She became the leading innovator in the field of what was then known as Radio–therapy, a most misleading term particularly in view of the rising popularity of the radio or wireless as it was called. Drown developed her own radionic instrument and called it the Homo–Vibra–Ray indicating that it employed the energies or life force of man's body in the course of diagnostic and treatment procedures. Nobody knows who decided to replace the human subject in the circuit with a metal detector plate covered with a rubber diaphragm, but replaced he was and Drown's instrument utilised a detector plate. Where Abrams had placed his patient's blood sample in the Dynamiser and percussed his subject's abdomen until he got a response, Drown gently stroked her fingers across the rubber diaphragm until a response was forthcoming. This response took the form of a 'stick' and a 'stick' was literally that — the operator's finger stuck to the rubber diaphragm when a positive reaction to a disease in the patient was recorded. I will deal with this in more detail further on in the book rather than go into details which could be confusing at this point.

One of Drown's most unusual discoveries was that treatment could be given from the diagnostic instrument at a distance. Like Abrams she had hooked her patients up to the instrument to give treatment. Of course she did not use the electro-magnetic energies that Abrams employed but instead circulated the life-force of the patient through the resistance dials and returned it to the patient's body modified by the rates set on the dials so that it would heal the disease.

Drown reasoned that we all live in a vast field of energy that surrounds the planet, and that we are in effect all connected by this field. If this was the case, she reasoned, then it should be possible, using the patient's blood sample as a link, to treat the patient at a distance. The moment she began this form of treatment which became known as 'broadcasting' she began getting results to support her assumptions. She could now both diagnose and treat at a distance.

To the average person this may sound far-fetched, but the fact is that it works. Drown, the remarkable woman that she was, went further. She invented a radionic camera which could take pictures of the insides of people although they were thousands of miles away at the time. It was logical to her. After all if everything shared one vast field of energy, then why not take pictures from a distance? Drown said that the blood spot of a patient was like a group of crystals and these crystals held the record of the whole person. By tuning the camera with a series of rates and placing the blood spot in the circuit, the film, which no light touched incidentally, would pick up the vibrations from the blood spot as selected by the rates, and impose an image on

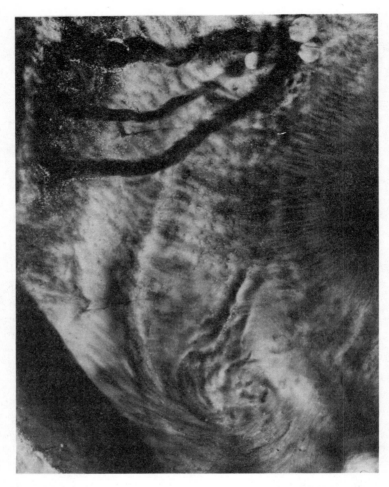

2. A radionic photograph taken during the 1930's by chiropractor, Ruth Drown, showing a cross-section of a human pelvis. The dark area in the bottom left-hand corner being the sacrum viewed side on. The tiny white dots which pervade the picture are bacteria and the three dark tube-like structures are blood vessels.

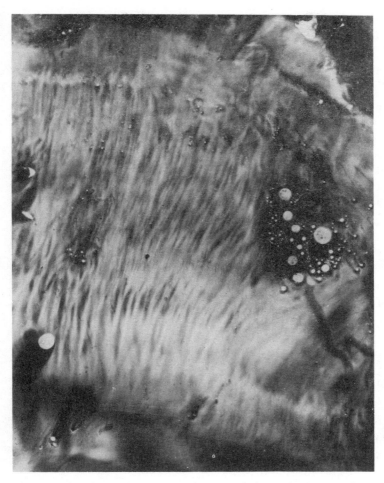

3. A Drown radionic photograph of a cyst in the liver of a patient. Where the camera picks up blood–vessels end on they appear as white discs.

the film. Scientifically this is impossible but Drown produced many hundreds of radionic photographs, and they are even more remarkable by virtue of the fact that these pictures of living human tissues bear an uncanny similarity to modern electron–microscope photographs.

While Drown ran her busy practice in Hollywood and continued to research the field of radionics, a growing number of doctors in England began to use radionic means as an aid to diagnosis, among them were such men as Dr. Dudley Wright, Dr. Eric Perkins, Dr. Winter Gonin, Dr. Guyon Richards and others. Of these Richards probably made the most significant contribution to radionics through his meticulous research work which is recorded in his book *The Chain of Life*. He also formed the Medical Society for the Study of Radiesthesia, of which radionics is a branch. This group was very active right into the 1970's, and put on many interesting lectures in London in order to promote this form of healing in the medical profession.

During the 1940's civil engineer, George De La Warr, began a serious investigation into radionics. Its theories and principles fascinated him and when he was approached by a practitioner with a request to build a replica of Drown's instrument he jumped at the chance, but not before asking her permission. As he studied the instrument he began to devise ways of improving upon it and eventually produced a more sophisticated diagnostic set which was to become very popular with practitioners, not only in England but throughout the world.

More and more of De La Warr's time became taken up by radionics, so that he left his post of Chief Engineering Assistant of the Oxfordshire County Council, and applied himself to radionic research on a full-time basis. Before long many research projects were initiated both in the agri-cultural and medical fields, and De La Warr's fertile mind conceived new forms of instrumentation. Marjorie, his wife, built a busy practice and earned a reputation as a first-class sensitive and diagnostician. She also compiled the books of rates used in the process of radionic diagnosis and treatment, and much of the success of the Laboratories was due to her skill as a healer. The De La Warrs were joined by Leonard Corte and instrument maker, Mr. Stevens, and these four formed the heart of the Laboratories. This period was probably the most intense in terms of radionic research, and, thanks to the efforts of the team, radionics became established in Britain. Today this country remains as un-challenged leader in the field of radionic healing, and doctors and health-care professionals from all over the world come here to study the latest procedures and developments.

It is way beyond the scope of this book to deal with all of the research that the De La Warr team carried out, or to discuss the multiplicity of instruments that were built and the ways in which they were employed to further our knowledge of radionics. Like Drown, George De La Warr developed a radionic camera which was used to take over 12,000 photographs of the energy fields of objects. Many of these photographs were unique; for example De La Warr took a blood spot from a pregnant woman and this was placed on the camera which was tuned to a three-month pregnancy. A film was slid into the light-tight box, left for 15 seconds, withdrawn, developed and printed. The image of a three-month-old foetus is very clear, and as a matter of interest the donor of the blood spot was over fifty miles from the camera when the picture was taken. It was phenomena like this that irritated the scientific community, and De La Warr's efforts to interest them in this work resulted for the most part in increased hostility. A doctor who had placed a radionic camera in a teaching hospital where he worked was told by the authorities in no uncertain terms to get it out, or they would both be removed from the premises.

By the 1960's radionics was well established in Britain,

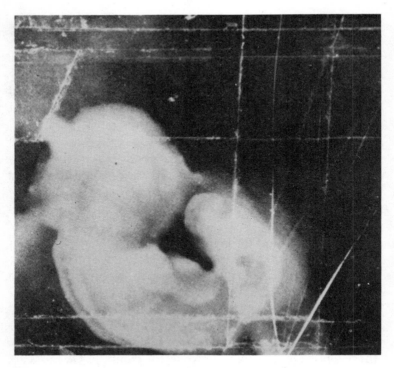

4. A radionic photograph taken at the De La Warr Laboratories in the 1950's. The image of the three month old foetus was obtained from the energies radiating from the blood spot of the mother, who was 54 miles from the camera when the picture was taken.

although in general it was practised by a relatively small number of people when one considers orthodox medicine or other healing arts. Nevertheless it had a strong following of patients from all walks of life, and you will see why as we get a little deeper into the subject.

For those who would like more details about radionics up to this point, I strongly recommend the two books written by George De La Warr and Langston Day entitled *New Worlds beyond the Atom* and *Matter in the Making*; both are excellent. For an overall and detailed outline of the full history of radionics there is no better book than *Report on Radionics* by Edward Russell.

I was introduced to radionics in 1967 by Dr. Aubrey Westlake, author of the popular book, *The Pattern of Health*, which deals with medical radiesthesia. Fascinated by what I saw I quickly joined the Radionic Association and began to study the subject. My training as a chiropractor gave me an excellent basis to work from during my studies, and to this was added my interest of many years standing, in the teachings of Eastern philosophy. At first glance the two may seem an odd combination, but in the teachings of the East man is always seen as a combination of inter-penetrating energy fields, and disease as a process of energy imbalances within these fields or energy bodies. In the ancient healing art of acupuncture for example, these principles are basic and disease is considered to be an imbalance of the life-force or 'chi' as it is called in China. There is an energy body comprised of meridians along which the life-force flows, and treatment with needles or moxa (burning) at specific points manipulates this life-force thus restoring health. Radionics, both from a diagnostic and treatment point of view, is tied up with the concept of a life-force.

What struck me as odd when I began my studies was that radionics was obviously a form of healing which dealt with energies of many kinds, but when I looked at the literature on the subject and the methods used in practice, the whole terminology and bias was towards the use of medical models of anatomy and pathology. This did not seem consistent to me; although I agreed with the fact that radionic diagnosis and treatment based on medical models worked, it did not seem to me that this approach even began to explore the real potential of radionics. With this in mind I began to correlate both Eastern and Western knowledge of man as energy rather than form, and to utilise concepts of Eastern subtle physiology and anatomy in my work. From these early researches came my first book *Radionics and the Subtle Anatomy of Man,* published in 1972. This book outlined a model of subtle bodies, called the etheric body — now often referred to as the bio-plasmic body — the emotional body and the mind, or mental body. Within these bodies were force centres or, as they are called in India and Tibet, the chakras. Through these vortices of energy certain energies flowed — too little or too much energy would upset the subtle bodies and ultimately create physical or psychological problems. It seemed logical to me that if disease manifested first at a subtle level before it became physical, then it would be in the patients' and the practitioners' interest if it could be identified at that level and treated before it became a real problem. Disease that had manifested would clear more quickly if tackled at the causative level where it originated. Subsequently this has proved to be the case, not only in radionics but in the more advanced forms of medical bio-electrical diagnosis.

Most practitioners soon took up the subtle body and chakra model and incorporated it into their practices because it extended their knowledge and capacity to pinpoint and treat the underlying causes of disease. The states of the chakras, as we shall later see, have a powerful bearing on our health from a physical and a psychological point of view. I will deal with this in more detail when I outline a radionic diagnosis.

Between 1972 and 1982 I wrote three more books on the subject, *Radionics — Interface with the Ether Fields, Dimensions of Radionics,* and *Radionics — Science or Magic?* These books in effect outline my researches in the field during this decade which has seen a growing interest in radionics by lay people and health-care professionals from many different disciplines. The books also details the vital work done in radionics by Malcolm Rae who I had the privilege of knowing and working with from time to time.

Malcolm Rae came from a diverse background of business and commerce, and like many others found that his interest in things unusual drew him into radionics and medical radiesthesia. He had an uncanny ability both as a practitioner and as a researcher to see things from many angles at once. Like every researcher in this field he sought to develop new and improved instruments and to refine techniques of diagnosis and treatment. Almost every week saw some new approach or idea emerge from his fertile mind during the 1970's. He incorporated the subtle anatomy and chakra analysis techniques, that I had developed, into his work, and I began using the new instruments he had developed in my practice. What emerged from the combining of our two approaches, forms today the essential basis of modern radionic techniques.

Apart from the new diagnostic instruments Rae developed, and the formulation of a new set of rates based on a 0 to 44 scale as opposed to the old 0 to 10, there was one outstanding contribution that has subsequently spread worldwide and is used by many medical doctors who practice homoeopathy, and that is the Potency Simulator. This small and apparently simple apparatus combined with specific geometric patterns can literally generate simulated homoeopathic medicines within the earth's magnetic field. Thus for example the remedy Arnica which is derived from the plant of that name, can be simulated with the instrument so accurately that the effect of the remedy made in the Simulator will be the same as that made from the plant. It was an outstanding contribution to the development of radionics and one which will continue to grow in this age of expanding awareness.

Obviously in a book of this size I cannot begin to cover the fascinating history of radionics in any great detail, but hopefully what I have outlined here will prompt you to take up further reading on the subject. As I go into other aspects of this healing art in the chapters to follow, you will find that the picture will begin to fill out. So far I have said little about radionic instruments, or just how a diagnosis is made at a distance, but we will come to that in good time.

3

Physical and Paraphysical Worlds

In order to really understand radionics it is essential to realise that all is energy! Now this is a statement with which physicists would agree, but they interpret it in ways that differ greatly from the vitalistic point of view. The vitalist sees a deep philosophical connotation in the words 'all is energy'! He sees spiritual meaning and purpose in these words because to him Life with a capital L is energy, and the more we come to understand things in terms of energy the closer we move towards the Source of all things, all life-forms.

Science recognizes that man has an electro–magnetic field which interpenetrates and surrounds his body and is distinct from the electro–magnetic field of the earth in which we and all life-forms live. This field can be measured with sensitive instruments such as a vacuum–tube voltmeter, and it can be influenced in various ways to either cause ill health, as, for example, by nuclear radiation, or, with electrical stimulus as used in certain acupuncture techniques, to improve health. Our electro–magnetic field is highly responsive to impacts of energy from the environment, and especially to directed thought as we shall see in a moment.

In the mid 1930's Dr. Saxton Burr put forward what he called the electro–dynamic theory of life. In this Burr posited that all physical forms, be they human, animal, vegetable or mineral, were held together and governed by underlying electro–magnetic fields of energy. Although these fields are invisible their action can be visualized by placing a magnet under a card and sprinkling iron filings over it. As the field exerts its influence the filings will be pulled into a pattern describing the lines of force of the magnetic field. The life-field, as it is called, is like a jelly-mould which produces a specific shape, and this shape or form is our physical body, which although separate from all other physical forms, is linked in terms of energy with other bodies. It is through this common energy-field that the radionic practitioner works when making a diagnosis and giving treatment from a distance.

Fluctuations in the earth's electro-magnetic field have a direct effect upon our vitality, and indeed our health in general. In the following extract from *Studies of Man in the Life-Field*, Dr. L. Ravitz, an expert in this area of medicine, describes how magnetic storms in space can affect us. He writes:

'One hot, humid June afternoon near new moon, two waitresses forget to serve their customers. Office help is drowsy and works perfunctorily. Elderly persons complain of profound lassitude. There is a large influx of new admissions on all hospital services with greatly increased birth and death rates — the latter pronounced during the afternoon hours — and patients begin to have markedly increased somatic symptoms. Almost half the psychiatric patients require increased supervision, and three are now suicidal. Certain abstinent alcoholics start to drink again, and crimes are rampant.

Two weeks later, the waitresses snap irritably at customers. Most of the office staff feel a 'second wind'. Another influx of hospital admissions occurs, but medical and surgical patients seem to have less intense symptoms. A different group of psychiatric patients is 'going into orbit', but none have been actively suicidal. Complaints of insomia are widespread, as are comments on unusually vivid dreams.'

This description by Dr. Ravitz is of course hypothetical, but these are the responses that occur when the electro-magnetic field we live in is subjected to intense disturbance. Medical science has made extensive studies of the earth's electro-magnetic field and careful monitoring has shown that there is a link between field flow and the strength and intensity of viral and bacterial epidemics. In short we are firmly locked into a life-field which links us all, and through this field distant effects can be seen to be caused.

The idea that energy fields lie beneath all physical forms is not by any means a new concept. Plato wrote of an archetypal essence which contained the predetermining images of the physical world. Paracelsus called it the Archeus and the ancient alchemists, the Nous. In Eastern philosophy the underlying energy field is called the etheric field and all physical forms are said to rise from it. Thus, in the Indian teachings, man is said to have an etheric body through which his physical body is vitalised and kept in a coherent state. According to the ancient sages the etheric body is composed of force currents, and in it are vital centres linked by lines of force with each other and the nervous system of the physical man. These lines of force connect man to the environing etheric system. The etheric body is vitalized and controlled by thought. So what this means in essence is that we are all connected and that there is no separation between any life-form on the etheric levels and the level of the mind. This provides the basis for distant healing and certainly for the biofeedback techniques that are now being utilised in holistic medicine whereby the patient is taught to control the body by thought, to reduce high temperatures, abort migraine headaches and in many instances to reverse the processes of terminal illness. The mind, when properly used, is all powerful in shaping health and harmony, and it is the trained mind that is utilised by the radionic practitioner. Once we understand this, the mystery goes out of radionics and we can begin to see how the practitioner can influence and improve the health of a distant patient.

In the early 1970's I had the privilege of working for a period with Marcel Vogel, chief research chemist for IBM in San Jose, California. This work involved man-plant communication experiments which demonstrated how plants responded to human thought. During the time I was with Marcel Vogel I witnessed some remarkable demonstrations of the power of thought on living systems. Prior to this, Marcel had measurably influenced a plant with three bursts of directed thought over a distance of six thousand miles. The response clearly showed on the strip-chart recorder which formed part of the instrumentation.

When Ruth Drown took radionic photographs she made use of the etheric field of the earth. Her theory was that the vital fluid-like force that pervaded everything could be manipulated in such a manner as to produce images on film. Drown made a profound statement when she said, "Everything *is here, now*. All we have to do is to tune in to it." We are so conditioned to seeings things in physical terms that it is hard for us to shift our way of perceiving. Certainly when we think in physical terms there is space between one person and another, but at the higher levels of consciousness this space is immediately eliminated by thought. Thus by thinking of a person you actually connect with them at that level; this is what Drown meant by 'everything *is here, now*. . .' and this is the basis of radionic work. When the practitioner tunes in with his mind to the patient, a linking immediately takes place and through this link the practitioner has access to information regarding the patient's health. Let us take a look now at how this process is utilised by the practitioner to make a radionic diagnosis. Later we will return to the subject of just how this process works, and look at it in a little more detail.

4

Your Radionic Analysis

You will note that the chapter heading says analysis and not diagnosis. This is because practitioners prefer to use the word analysis, firstly because an analysis is made of the patient's state of health in terms that are not strictly medical. Diagnosis is a medical term and a doctor does diagnose, he tells you, by name, the disease you have. A radionic practitioner on the other hand is seeking to determine a more holistic picture of your health status under a number of different categories and in this manner analyses the states of the various aspects of your physical and paraphysical bodies. Above all he looks for the causative factor or factors that lie behind your illness, because these will determine the treatment required by you as an individual.

Most people are introduced to radionics through a friend or relative, or they read a book on the subject and become interested in it in this manner. Let us assume you have written to or telephoned a radionic practitioner in order to seek his or her help with a health problem. You will be asked to fill in a case-history form, giving details of your past medical history, listing accidents, surgery, past illnesses and, in particular, childhood diseases such as measles, mumps, chicken-pox and so forth. You will also be asked to list any drugs you have taken, or may presently be taking, in both a medical or recreational sense. And some details may be requested regarding diseases suffered by your parents and grandparents. To this can be added any other relevant data plus details of your present problem and symptoms.

The completed form is then returned to the practitioner with a snippet of your hair, which should be placed in an envelope with your name on it. Practitioners normally supply these along with the case-history form. Your snippet of hair is known as the 'witness' and it serves as a link between you and the practitioner while he is making the analysis, during treatment, or at any time your progress needs to be monitored.

Having received your details the practitioner will study your past and current health problems to familiarise himself with your condition. This in effect is a part of the process of tuning into you at a distance. Next an Analysis Sheet is prepared with your name, address and details on it. This is set to one side while the practitioner then prepares your 'witness'. This is done by taking a small amount of hair, placing it between two tacky discs of paper, and carefully printing your name on it for purposes of identification. The practitioner is now ready to make your radionic analysis.

Before I go into any details regarding the analysis or diagnostic procedure, I think we should consider the instrument used for this purpose. There are in fact many different designs, so I propose to outline the basic components of the average radionic instrument. It consists of a box some 18 inches x 14 inches and 4 inches deep, and usually has a panel covering the top made from black perspex. As a rule there are twelve dials set in rows of four, the first of which is calibrated from 0 to 100; the remaining eleven are calibrated 0 to 10. Frequently there is one other dial set on its own; this is the measuring dial used for measuring the intensity or levels of diseases, toxins and so forth and like the first dial it is calibrated from 0 to 100. Next there is a well to hold the 'witness' during the analysis, or instead of a well there may be a chromed metal disc to put the 'witness' on. Then there may be a rotatable magnet and finally a detector plate. In some sets this is nothing more than the chrome disc already mentioned, or it may be a

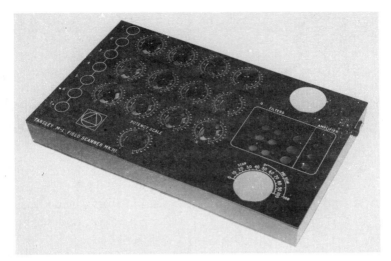

5. Tansley M–L Field Scanner Mk III radionic diagnostic instrument, which is used for distant diagnosis and treatment.

more elaborate affair with a rubber diaphragm stretched tightly across it. Beneath the top panel of the instrument, the dials are connected to potentiometers the same as those used in a radio. These are usually wired in series to the well and the detector plate so that a circuit is formed along which the energy patterns from the 'witness' can travel.

I mentioned earlier that Dr. Abrams had determined numerical values for all disease conditions, organs of the body, chemicals, toxins and in fact anything that was relevant to this form of diagnosis or analysis. These have been expanded, developed and modified over the years, but in short these numerical values are known as 'rates' and they serve to identify and represent symptoms, diseases, organs and so forth. All disease rates begin with a double digit; for example, fractured ribs have an identification rate of 90.7542, hence the calibration of the first dial on the instrument — known as the 'disease dial' — of 0 to 100. If the practitioner were to use this rate to determine the presence of fractured ribs, he would put 90 on the first dial setting and then 7, 5, 4 and 2 on subsequent dials. If on the other hand he wanted to measure the functional integrity of a part of the body, say the ligaments, he would leave the first dial at 0 and place the rate of 854 on the next three dials. Setting the dials in this manner provides a stabilising frequency of the body part or disease in question, and enables the practitioner to concentrate on making the analysis.

When you submitted your details you would have listed your present symptoms. The practitioner will select one of these upon which to base the analysis. How does he do this? Well this brings us to the point where I will have to describe the process through which the practitioner can detect and identify disease patterns at a distance. There are basically two methods; the oldest one utilises the detector plate with the rubber diaphragm stretched over it. Having placed your 'witness' in the well of the instrument, with all of the dials set at 0, the practitioner will stroke the diaphragm and at the same time he will begin to rotate the magnet slowly; in his mind he asks for the critical rotational position of the magnet in relationship to the magnetic field of the earth. His fingers will sweep across the diaphragm from right to left with ease until the magnet comes into the right position. When the 'stick' occurs the practitioner knows that the magnet is in its critical rotational position, which means it is in a position to stabilise all of the energies within the instrument during the analysis work. There is evidence too, suggesting that the magnet helps to stabilise the energy fields of the practitioner during his work, thus offsetting fatigue.

Having done this the next step is to apply the same process to the list of your symptoms. Stroking the diaphragm with the fingers of his right hand, the left is used to point a stylus at each symptom in turn, while mentally asking, "Is this the correct symptom to be used for the analysis?" The moment the right symptom is pointed at the 'stick' will occur. The rate for that symptom is straight away put up on the dials of the instrument. The practitioner then, in a methodical manner, using the same process over and over again, determines which organ systems are involved in the symptom. Then these organs are broken down into sub-divisions or the specific parts of the organ affected. Having done this the practitioner seeks out the causes for the imbalances in each organ and its sub-divisions. These causes may range from viral infection, bacteria, poisons, food additives, hormone imbalances, mineral deficiencies, or toxins left over from childhood diseases. Often psychological factors are identified, such as anger, fear or anxiety, and all are listed to form an analysis of your health. Having determined the causes of your illness, the practitioner then finds out what treatment is required. If there are aspects of your condition that are best dealt with by a practitioner from another healing discipline, then it will be suggested that you contact the appropriate person. If not, then radionic treatment will be initiated. I will deal with this process in a later chapter.

Now I mentioned earlier that there were two different methods of detecting disease radiations and I have described the way the 'stick pad' technique works. The other method, and the one most commonly employed today, is to use a pendulum which is swung over the 'witness' placed on the chrome metal disc or detector plate of the instrument. The same principle applies in that, as the pendulum swings back and forth over the 'witness', the practitioner mentally asks one question after another. For example he may mentally ask, "Are measles toxins present in this patient?" If they are, the pendulum will begin to rapidly swing in a clockwise direction by way of answering yes. If not, then the pendulum continues to oscillate back and forth. In reality the practitioner is dowsing for disease just as some people dowse for water or lost objects. It is a process that can also

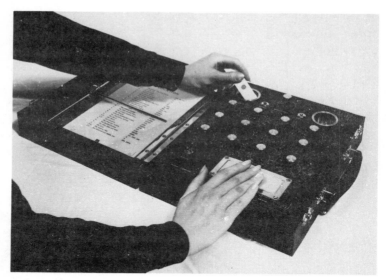

6. Patient's 'witness' (blood spot or snippet of hair) being introduced into a De La Warr diagnostic instrument while detector pad is being stroked to elicit a reaction or 'stick'.

be employed to find out which foods we are allergic to. This form of dowsing for disease and for the correct selection of homoeopathic remedies was popularised by a number of French priests in the 1930's, and the most famous of these was the Abbé Mermet, whose book *Principles and Practice of Radiesthesia* was published in 1935. In the same year Mermet's work and researches, and those of his colleagues, received the Paternal Blessing of the Pope.

The foregoing gives a broad picture of the process of radionic analysis technique. We can sum it up by saying that the practitioner tunes into you, the patient at a distance, using his mind with the radionic instrument serving as a focus to work through. There are as many techniques, if not more, as there are types of instrument. Radionic diagnostic work is very personal and every practitioner, although he or she may follow a basic outline, has his or her own particular

method. This being the case I think, for purposes of clari-
fication, it will help if I outline the approach and procedure
that I employ in practice, and follow this up by illustrating a
typical analysis and giving the interpretation of findings.

First I assess the Vitality Index using a scale of 0 to 100 to
measure against. A reading of 75 is average, 80 to 85 is ideal.
70 or below indicates that there is a real imbalance in the
body at some point or another. Next the Physical Health
and Psychological Health Indices are measured on the same
scale. By comparing these two readings some insight is
gained into the nature of the problem, as to whether it is
predominantly physical in nature or psychosomatic. For
example, a patient listing many symptoms, yet having an
average or better than average Physical Health Index but a
low Psychological one, most likely is ill as a result of
emotional and psychological stresses. On the other hand a
good Psychological Health Index and a poor Physical one
would point towards more physical causes. These figures
initially provide the basic guide to the state of the patient as
outlined above, and during treatment and at the cessation of
treatment the new measurements will indicate progress
towards normal.

The next stage is to determine and measure the functional
and structural integrity of the organ systems of the body,
and to ascertain if they are over or under–active. The scale
once again is 0 to 100, and in this instance 0 represents
optimum health of the organ and 100 the maximum
deviation from optimum health. By measuring each organ
system and entering the reading on the Analysis Sheet, a
picture begins to emerge, and I mean quite literally that,
because the state of the organs shows up graphically on the
chart, their deviation from normal being plotted by a graph
line which is drawn from one point to another. It is
important to realise that these readings are based on the
energy state of the organ concerned. So if a particularly
poor reading on an organ is indicated, it may not mean that

the organ is necessarily physically distressed. However if an organ's energy field has been in a state of high imbalance for a long period of time, the chances are that there may be cellular degeneration.

Having measured each organ system, the next factor that is checked is the possible presence of toxins. Now toxins may be stored in various cells of the body and may take the form of residues left over from childhood diseases, or they may come from chemical sources such as insecticides from working in the garden or under industrial conditions. Food additives and preservatives can also lodge in our cells and create toxic conditions in the gut. Medical drugs and anti-biotics likewise pollute cellular structures in such a way that the organ where they lodge never really works at an optimum level as long as they are there. There are many different toxic factors that we are subjected to, often unwittingly, so I shall deal with these in a later chapter.

Having established if there are toxins present the next step is to determine if any miasms are imbedded in the physical and etheric matrix of the body. Miasm is the name given to a specific focus or pattern of energy which will predispose you to certain diseases and symptoms. The concept of the miasm arose out of the work of Hahnemann who founded the healing art of homoeopathy. Miasms, it seems, can be inherited or acquired and it is not uncommon to find, say, a tubercular miasm in a patient, and upon pointing this out to them they will then recall that their father once contracted the disease or a grandparent had in fact died from it many years previously. It seems that in some way or other the predisposition is passed from one generation to another genetically, and may simply remain quiescent unless the individual leads a life that encourages these seeds of disease to germinate and finally turn into a recognizable clinically identifiable disease. Clearly if these disease patterns can be handed down from one generation to the next, it is important to break this causal chain through the appropriate treatment.

What has been considered so far? Your level of vitality, and the guideline measurements of your physical and psychological health. The organ systems have been checked for their levels of structural and functional integrity and the measurements of these noted on your chart. The presence of toxins and miasms has been carefully determined and their intensity measured and recorded. Apart from identifying psychological causative factors that might be present, this analysis would be virtually complete according to the procedures used by practitioners prior to 1972. In 1972, when I introduced the concept of the chakras and the subtle anatomy in *Radionics and the Subtle Anatomy of Man,* a new method of analysis was inaugurated, which enabled practitioners to determine deeper and more fundamental causes of dis-ease. We shall look at these in a moment.

The beauty of radionics is that it works at all levels and caters to all people who are open-minded enough to be able to accept its principles. In this manner a radionic analysis that deals with physical organ systems and diseases, using what is essentially a medical model of anatomy, physiology and pathology, can in itself be seen as a 'complete' system. There are many people who can accept this level of analysis, but who would be totally mystified and put off by such terms as the chakras and subtle anatomy. Accepting these new concepts is more of a quantum leap in awareness than some individuals are prepared to make, which is fair enough. Some people do not want to know about the more philosophical and esoteric causes of their condition. If John Doe has varicose veins, he may not be interested in the subtleties of chakra imbalance as it applies to his condition. To him a varicose vein is a varicose vein, it hurts and he wants to get rid of the problem, and that's it as far as he is concerned.

Today however there is a large and growing legion of patients who want to look deeper into themselves, and to come to a fuller understanding of their condition. They may for example, want to gain some insight into the psychological and spiritual aspects of their dis-ease, even if it is something as apparently mundane as a chronically stiff neck. Knowledge of the chakras and the subtle anatomy enables the radionic practitioner to meet this need and demand, and as the depth of his or her knowledge increases, the capacity to heal will be extended and broadened. Healing a patient does not always mean getting rid of the symptoms; often it means helping them to adopt a different attitude to their condition, so that they learn from the experience rather than exhausting themselves, and perhaps the practitioner, in fighting the dis-ease.

If you are a patient who wants deeper knowledge of your condition, then it is essential that your radionic analysis deals with the chakras. As we have already seen the concept of centres of energy and energy bodies underlying our physical form is to be found in virtually all philosophical and religious belief systems throughout the world. Many of us are aware of the fact that acupuncture is based on a system of meridians and acupuncture points which can be measured with electrical instrumentation. Acupuncture points are in effect tiny chakras or centres of force along the meridians, through which 'chi', the life-force flows. In Tibetan and Indian medicine the life-force is called 'prana' and it flows through a series of much larger vortices of energy known as the chakras, as well as many smaller centres including the acupuncture points.

There are seven major chakras located in the energy field along the cerebro-spinal axis, and they are not in any sense physical although they relate directly to the various nerve plexi and especially to the endocrine glands. Each chakra governs certain areas of the physical body by way of the etheric or bio-plasmic body which supports and vitalises it.

Although it is a highly complex system, the fundamental principles are quite simple in that according to the Indian priest-physicians of ancient times, our body depends in great measure on the proper flow of various energies through the chakras to the nervous system, the endocrine glands and the organs of the body. If this flow is too strong, erratic or too weak, then disease can eventuate. Like Dr. Abrams, they are stating that disease is a matter of energy imbalance rather than cellular in origin. The following chart will clarify the relationship between the chakras, the glands and the organs of the body.

It becomes clear that if there is an imbalance in the way a chakra is functioning, and the practitioner is only concerned with the physical systems of the body, then he is going to miss the fundamental cause of the dis-ease. For example in many cases of asthma the throat chakra is damaged; if this damage is not dealt with the asthma will remain and require fairly constant medication of one kind or another. It is logical that if the practitioner treats the chakra to normalise its function by radionic means, then the asthma is far more likely to clear.

When a radionic practitioner analyses the states of the chakras he looks for underactivity and overactivity, and he looks for blockages to the flow of energy through the chakra. An underactive chakra indicates as a rule that the patient is suppressing the flow of energy through a chakra, and an overactive chakra shows that too much energy is being directed through the chakra. To give an example of how this affects the individual let us look at the solar plexus chakra which is a common cause of dis-ease. The solar plexus chakra externalises as the pancreas and governs the stomach, liver, gall bladder and sympathetic nervous system. Apart from the physical role it has to play each chakra deals with energies that are concerned with mental, intellectual and emotional functions. This being the case, and the fact that the solar plexus chakra is the seat of desire

The Seven Major Spinal Chakras

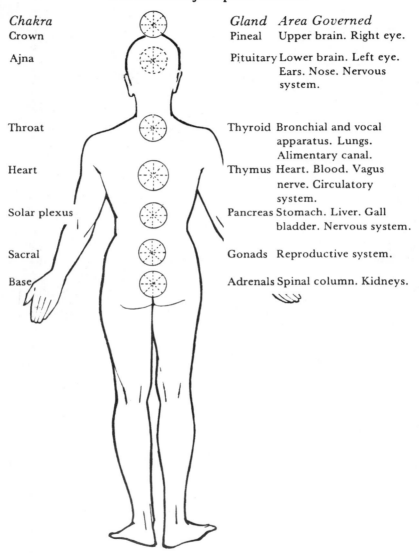

Chakra	Gland	Area Governed
Crown	Pineal	Upper brain. Right eye.
Ajna	Pituitary	Lower brain. Left eye. Ears. Nose. Nervous system.
Throat	Thyroid	Bronchial and vocal apparatus. Lungs. Alimentary canal.
Heart	Thymus	Heart. Blood. Vagus nerve. Circulatory system.
Solar plexus	Pancreas	Stomach. Liver. Gall bladder. Nervous system.
Sacral	Gonads	Reproductive system.
Base	Adrenals	Spinal column. Kidneys.

7. The chakras, or force centres, which govern the human form, the mind and the emotional states.

and emotion, we have in its over or underactivity a potent source of trouble. If emotions and desires are suppressed and their energies not expressed properly through the solar plexus chakra then diseases of the pancreas, liver and gall bladder are most likely to occur. If the predisposition towards cancer is in the patient then the suppressed energy will eventually build itself a tumor to express itself. People who are highly emotional often have overactive solar plexus chakras, they too are subject to various diseases of the related organs, and the sympathetic nervous system becomes highly overactive and can lead to various psychological problems.

The ajna, or brow chakra, presents us with another interesting insight as to the importance of the chakras in a radionic analysis. The brow chakra as the name suggests is located in the region of the forehead, it externalises as the pituitary gland and governs the sinuses, teeth, ears, eyes and brain stem. This important chakra is also known as the centre of the personality, thus an individual who has an overactive brow chakra will tend to be extroverted and highly motivated towards achieving success in life. They are frequently over-strivers and perfectionists who put a lot of energy into whatever they are doing. On the other hand if this chakra is underactive you may have an introverted, withdrawn type of person, who never really express themselves. While the former is more likely to suffer migraine headaches the latter gets bogged down in sinus and catarrhal conditions and may have poor eyesight as well. The pituitary which is the conductor of the endocrine 'orchestra' is a vitally important gland and plays an important role in the female menstrual cycle. An imbalance in the brow chakra can often result in pre-menstrual tension and periods combined with migraine headaches.

From these brief details it will begin to become clear that the chakras play an important role in our physical and psychological health, so by including them in his radionic analysis the practitioner is encompassing deeper causes of dis-ease which may well have been previously incorrectly ascribed to more physical factors.

Of course the practitioner cannot analyse the state of the chakras without taking into consideration the subtle bodies. I have mentioned them earlier on in the book, and they are the etheric — or vital bio-plasmic body — which is the densest subtle body; next is the emotional, or astral body as it is sometimes called. It is in this body that we experience the various emotional energies and have the focus of our desire-life. Anger, fear, depression or the desire for a new hi-fi or car are all qualities of astral energy which sweep through this body, galvanising it into activity. It is closely linked to the solar plexus chakra, and as I previously mentioned this is a potent source of disease. Finally there is the mental body through which our intellectual and cognitive processes work. Thought involves the use of the mental body, and it enables us to discriminate and apply logical processes to the running of our lives.

Like the chakras these bodies are subject to problems which the practitioner has to consider. Each of the bodies may for example become congested. Mental congestion usually consists of half-formed unclear thoughts which mount up like piles of rubbish in the mental body and prevent clear thinking. Unexpressed desires and emotions can similarly cloud the emotional body, and at a more physical level, lack of exercise and sunshine, or excesses of junk foods clog up the etheric body causing congestion. Each body can also become over-stimulated and this can lead to a variety of dis-ease states. Finally there is the condition known as lack of coordination; this can occur between the mental and emotional bodies, between the emotional body and the etheric, or more commonly between the etheric and the physical form. When the etheric body is not properly linked into the physical you have an individual who tends towards frailty in extreme cases or just plain chronic fatigue if they have a reasonably normal physical body.

By now you will begin to have an inkling just how comprehensive a radionic analysis can be, and it must at this point be becoming obvious just how this technique can really probe deeply beyond symptom patterns to the causes of disease which inevitably lie hidden at some level or another of our being. What I have outlined so far — that is the analysis of the organ systems, the chakras and the subtle bodies — is what should be covered in an analysis made by most practitioners today. I should stress, however, as I have said earlier, that each radionic practitioner follows his or her own system and that not all practitioners use this system of analysis and treatment. If you are in any doubt it would be wise to enquire before you request analysis and treatment from a practitioner. There are even deeper aspects but I will reserve them for a separate chapter further on in the book. Let us go now to the interpretation of an analysis that has been made, the substance of which, along with a copy of the chart, would come as a report to you, the patient.

5

Radionic Analysis Interpretation

Interpretation of a radionic analysis is clearly an art which should involve the intuitive abilities of the practitioner, based on his knowledge of the various aspects of the method he or she uses. As I pointed out in the previous chapter this may be along medical lines, in which case the chakras and subtle bodies will not be included. But for the purposes of this chapter, and due to the fact that most practitioners now take the more subtle elements into consideration I will include them.

The interpretation comes to you, the patient, in the form of a report. It may be brief and to the point, taking up a few lines, or it may cover as many as four or five foolscap pages, in which case it becomes somthing more than a report, and serves to express a form of guidance as to the way you are handling or mis-handling energies, and how this is affecting your health. This can be an important factor in the report because dis-ease is a matter of too much or too little energy in any given area of the body. If you can be made aware of just what is going on, then you can begin to take a more active and constructive role in the improvement and maintenance of your health. We live in a 'fix it' society, we drive our car in to be fixed, we get the TV fixed or the washing machine fixed. This attitude is too often applied to health — people walk into their doctor's office with a 'fix me' attitude, and they get treated that way with a drug prescription that often makes them sicker than they already were. As a rule the radionic practitioner expects to educate

Vitality Index 70			Name JOHN DOE		Date 15-1-84
Physical Health Index 74 Psychological Health Index 75			Address FAIRLAWN, HIGHWAY, THORPE, SY.		
Congestion ETHERIC 50.			Birth Date 25 Day 1 Month 50 Year		LONDON. Place
Over-Stimulation ASTRAL 60. ETHERIC 55.			Symptoms FATIGUE. INDIGESTION.CATARRH.		
Lack of Co-ordination ETHERIC 30.			Miasms —	Toxins MEASLES 60	

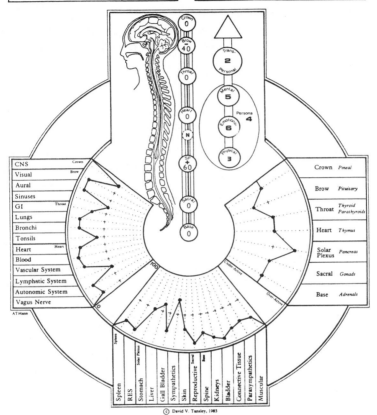

8. A radionic analysis chart showing the states of the organ systems, the chakras and the ray energies which condition the subtle bodies and, ultimately, the physical form.

his patient in the ways of health, and the analysis report
serves as the basis for his advice along these lines.

I think the best way in which this analysis chart can be
explained is for me to write a report to a hypothetical John
Doe in response to his request for a radionic analysis. We
will assume that he has a basic knowledge of the chakras and
subtle anatomy, and is not unfamiliar with the terminology
I will use.

Dear Sir,
I have recently heard about radionics from a friend who has
received much benefit from radionic treatment, and I wondered if
you would be so kind as to take me on as a patient. My main
problems are chronic fatigue and catarrh for which I have tried all
kinds of treatment to little avail. Please find enclosed my case
history and a small lock of hair. I hope that you will be able to help
me and I look forward to hearing from you soon.

Yours sincerely
John Doe

Dear John Doe,
Thank you for your letter requesting a radionic analysis and the
enclosed details of your medical health history and current
symptoms.

The analysis indicates a Vitality Index of 70 which is low, but in
keeping with your feeling of chronic fatigue. 75 is an average
reading and 80 ideal. Your Physical and Psychological Health
Indices are about average at 74 and 75 respectively. Your spleen
chakra is functioning normally so your etheric body is taking in
and distributing prana properly. So it is the way you are utilising
your energies which is resulting in fatigue. This will become
more clear as I continue.

You have a fairly high level of congestion in your etheric body,
suggesting perhaps improper diet and a lack of proper exercise.
There is a high reading on over-stimulation of your emotional
body, indicating that you are in a somewhat tense state, and this
of course is being reflected into the etheric body and further
depleting your energy. Compounding the problem is a lack of
coordination between your etheric and physical bodies; this
always leads to depletion and in some cases gives the ability to

function mediumistically, not something, in the circumstances, which should be encouraged.

You have a high level of measles toxins in your central nervous system, or to be more precise, the meninges of the brain. This is yet another factor which may be contributing to your fatigued state and may well give you a feeling of muzziness in the head and a lack of clarity in your thinking processes.

Looking at your organ systems on the chart the central nervous system shows a reading of 50; this irritation as I have mentioned already is due to the measles toxin, a disease you contracted in childhood. The organ systems by the way are measured on an arbitrary scale of 0 to 100. The 0 represents optimum health of a system and 100 the maximum deviation from the optimum. Please don't forget that these are energy readings, so a poor reading does not necessarily mean actual physical changes have taken place in the organs showing poor readings. Many of these change rapidly towards normal when treated, those that lag behind are usually the focus of trouble. Any reading of 30 indicates a significant imbalance, so your important readings are Central Nervous System 50. Sinuses 50. Tonsils 40. Lymphatics 50. Stomach 50. Liver 60. and Sympathetic Nervous System 70.

The Central Nervous System and tonsil readings are related to the measles toxin and so in part is the lymphatic reading, as they try to deal with this when it becomes more active; which is when you get stressed for periods of time, and particularly if you are involved in a lot of mental activity at work.

To look a little deeper into your health problem we must consider the chakras. Of the seven major force centres, you have two that are out of balance. The first is the brow chakra; this centre relates directly to the pituitary gland and governs the sinuses, ears, eyes, teeth and the lower brain. The fact that your brow chakra is underactive indicates that you tend to repress your personality and never really fully express yourself. This results in congestion, not to mention frustration and is partly responsible for your chronic catarrh. You are blocking energies at that level, so there is a need to learn to express yourself more fully. You should note that both your visual and aural readings of 10 reflect this block to some extent.

The other chakra that is out of balance is the solar plexus centre which is situated just below the diaphragm. It is related to the pancreas and governs your liver, gall bladder and stomach. While its overactivity is having a minimal effect upon your gall bladder, both the liver and stomach are reacting adversely to the stress placed upon them. Likewise your whole sympathetic nervous system is on edge and tensed up due to the excessive amount of energy coming through this area. It indicates that you are far too emotional in your responses to life and everyday situations in general. You function through your feeling nature rather than through mental comprehension, and this places a lot of strain on your nervous system, and the hyper-activity of your emotional body further depletes your vitality. You can perhaps realise too that the overactive desire and emotional aspect of your life is in a sense frustrated because your personality often fails to put ideas into action.

In practical terms you need to learn to be more outgoing as an individual, and express yourself in small ways at first. Do this deliberately and note your successes; also never let failure deter you, keep at it. Closing down your solar plexus and quietening your emotional body can be accomplished by the age old method of counting to ten before you react to a given situation. Look at things logically and as they are, not as you *feel* about them. This is not a matter of *repressing feeling,* for that can be dangerous, but *transmuting* and *transforming* it to a higher level of cognizance.

You will feel a lot better once the measles toxins are cleared from your central nervous system, and as the treatment helps you to balance the activities of the brow and solar plexus chakras, the organ systems they govern will begin to settle down. The under-active reading on your muscular system suggests that proper exercise would not go amiss. Make sure your diet is balanced, avoid excessive intake of tea or coffee, the former will give you dyspepsia and the latter is an adrenal stimulant and will throw even more strain upon your nervous system. I suggest that you boil the herb Rosemary and strain the liquid into your bath water, this will help to bring the etheric body into a better relationship to the physical.

This, then, is how a report would read. There are of course other details which could be added but, as you can see, in general it gives the patient a deeper insight into his or her health problem than a standard radionic report would, and it puts the ball back into the patient's court to some extent by pointing out what they need to do in the way of major shifts of attitude and the use of their energies. This is a simple example but even so it would require a patient with some real self-knowledge to grasp all of its implications. Of course not all patients have this deeper grasp of more esoteric matters, in which case the straight forward report is indicated and the problem is outlined in the more familiar medical terms.

You may have noticed the series of circles with the triangle on top, and some numbers on this chart. The circles represent the subtle bodies and are marked accordingly, the ovoid represents the personality or combined energies of the mental, emotional and etheric bodies. The numbers relate to specific qualities of energy which give rise to definite character traits. I will deal with this aspect of radionic analysis in a separate chapter because it is a peculiarly specialised form of analysis and is only of use to patients who have a background in this area of inter-pretation.

It is clear even from this brief outline that a radionic analysis looks beyond symptoms for the causes of disease, and it is these causes that it treats when seeking to heal a patient.

6

Radionic Treatment

Today the term 'holistic' is bandied about in healing circles to such a degree that even orthodox medicine is laying claim to it. An holistic approach to health and healing implies that the whole person is seen and treated as a complex psycho-somatic organism, pervaded by the power of the trans-personal self or soul. If you look at many of the so called holistic therapies currently in vogue, it immediately becomes apparent that their concept of holism is to bunch several already accepted forms of treatment which are primarily physically oriented, into one lump, and call this holistic healing. This in truth is not an holistic approach. Holism not only requires that the patient be seen as a spiritual–psycho–somatic being, but that the therapist too is aware of his own holism. Only in this manner can he or she approach the patient in a holistic manner. In other words the practitioner approaches the problems of the patient in terms of the whole person, seeking the inner causes of disease, not only in generally accepted terms but in the complex interactions of energy between the various components of the subtle bodies with the physical form, and in the dynamic activity of the chakras. If any therapy can claim to be holistic, then it is radionics. As you will see, radionic treatment approaches every patient and every health problem as unique.

It should be evident by now that the radionic method of diagnosis has many advantages over orthodox clinical techniques. I am not about to decry the latter, for the simple reason that any approach that enables practitioners to bring help to their patients is valid. In a physically oriented society, physical methods are required and have their place. However, as I have previously stated there is a vast number of people today who are not satisfied with orthodox methods, who take advantage of the fact that a radionic analysis penetrates beyond the physical levels to ascertain the true and hidden causes of illness. They are aware that a swiftly scribbled prescription for drugs is in most instances nothing more than a suppressive measure that leaves the cause of their trouble untouched.

Physical diagnosis clearly has physical limitations, but in the hands of a highly skilled radionic practitioner, a radionic diagnostic instrument can be used to lay out the whole inner map, or health blueprint of the individual. This blueprint provides the basis for radionic treatment. Dr. Saxton Burr showed in his medical researches into the human energy field that any distortion of the field will eventually manifest as dis-ease. Radionic analysis work determines the nature and location of disturbed and disturbing energies within the paraphysical fields, and then treats these distortions with the appropriate 'rates' or energy frequencies. It is beyond the scope of this book to go into all the technicalities involved in radionic treatment, but a general outline can be given which should clarify what must seem a rather curious, even mysterious, process to some people.

As we have seen energy fields underlie and connect all life-forms, and distant events such as solar magnetic storms in space affect us here on earth. There are many research projects involving the study of distant effects, few find exposure through the media. How many people for example know that it is a medically documented fact that blood clotting time in patients undergoing surgery is affected by the phases of the moon? Very few I would imagine. One of the most publicised events concerning **distant influencing was when astronaut Edgar Mitchell** carried out experiments in telepathy during his historic flight to the moon. His revelation to the press regarding the nature of these experiments unleashed a great flurry of interest and activity. It then came to light that a great deal of experimentation in distant influencing and allied areas was going on in Russia. Thus it was that a new era in parapsychology began to blossom in the late 1960's and has continued to expand ever since.

Of course action and influence at a distance as employed in radionic treatment is nothing new and has been an integral part of folk lore and folk medicine since the dawn of time. The famed physician Paracelsus, whose alchemical works gave much impetus to modern chemistry, firmly believed in the concept of action at a distance. He wrote:

The sun can shine through a glass, and fire can radiate warmth through the walls of a stove, although the sun does not pass through the glass and the fire does not go through the stove; *in the same way, the human body can act at a distance while remaining at rest in one place.*

This is a remarkable statement, but other men of science and extraordinary intellectual ability like Leibnitz, Kant and Sir Isaac Newton have debated the phenomena of action at a distance, and today more and more evidence is accumulating to show that it is a reality. I dealt with this at some length in my book *Radionics — Interface with the Ether Fields,* and I do not think I can do better than to draw on that material to illustrate radionic treatment. In *Interface* I pointed out that the work of Backster and Vogel had established that plants and other life forms have a definite and sympathetic response to what is happening in their environment; and further that their experiments had shown that action at a distance — long ascribed to gravitational forces originating in planets — was in fact a feature of a less material field of energy which tallies with the etheric body of the earth and its response to thought, as described in the ancient Vedas of India.

To the radionic practitioner who treats patients at a distance every day, and sees the constructive and healing effects of this work, action at a distance, so hotly debated in scientific circles, is an everyday phenomenon. To the orthodox and less flexible mind such techniques seem highly suspect, yet in the sixteenth and seventeenth centuries the sympathetic cure of wounds was a well authenticated happening.

In his *Sylva Sylvarum,* published in 1672, Francis Bacon wrote: "It is constantly received and avouched, that the anointing of the weapon that maketh the wound, will heal the wound itself." He then described the preparation of an ointment, and the various tests to which the practice has been subjected, all of which seem to show that the cure is obtained only when the ointment is applied to the weapon and not to the wound, that the weapon may be at a great distance, and that the cure does not depend on the patient knowing of the anointing.

There is a clear parallel here to radionic treatment. Bacon states that the healing ointment is placed upon the sword that made the wound, and we assume that the patient's witness in the form of blood is on the blade. Thus the healing agent is brought into proximity with a part of the patient — his blood that stains the blade. In radionic treatment the hair witness serves the same purpose, and is subjected to the healing frequencies of various radionic rates, thus affecting the patient at a distance; at least this is the view held by many practitioners.

Sir Kenelm Digby was famous for his work in distant healing, and had a version of the cure in which a cloth covered with blood from the wound is soaked in a solution of the 'Powder of Sympathy' (specially prepared from iron sulphate). Glanville asserted that the cure of wounds at a distance had been put out of all doubt by the noble Sir Digby.

In Spratt's *History of the Royal Society,* a writer remarks that a reported effect on wounds of a certain poison from Macassar, which touches the blood from the wound, is not strange to those who study sympathy. Many years ago it was recorded that Suffolk ploughmen would similarly treat objects that had inflicted wounds on horses, thus healing the animal by distant means. How then does this all tie in with radionics?

Healing at a distance depends on a field of energy in which the patient and the practitioner are submerged. Both practitioner and patient have their own distinct energy fields, but these can be linked with each other by an act of thought. Science knows a great deal about what fields do and their effects but it really does not know what they are. Radionics utilises the fact that we are all inextricably linked by one vast field of energy; radio and television utilise different levels of the same field to transmit words, music and pictures. When we really stop to think about the fact that a picture can be drawn from the apparently empty space of your living room, that has been transmitted from the other side of the world, or even from outer space, it causes no eyebrows to be raised. But the minute you state that a practitioner using radionic instruments can diagnose and heal at a distance there is, more often than not, objection. There shouldn't be, because the practitioner merely makes use of different levels of the same energy field. The fact that science does not yet fully recognize them (although it is being forced in this direction) does not mean that these levels do not exist, nor that they cannot be used for purposes of diagnosis and treatment of disease.

Having said all this, what does the practitioner do when he or she gives radionic treatment? Well, treatment takes a number of forms and there are various procedures and types of treatment instruments — some use geometric patterns on cards, others employ the radionic rates or numbers. I will describe the use of a standard radionic treatment instrument which comprises of an upright box some 10″ long, 7″ high

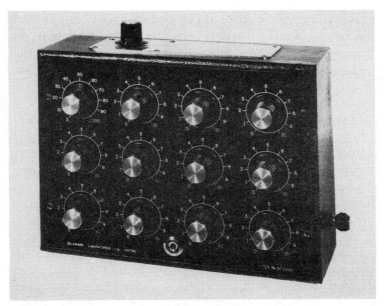

9. A De La Warr radionic treatment set. Specific rates or numerical treatment values are placed on the dials to treat the patient at a distance. The patient's 'witness' is placed on the metal plate on top of the instrument, and flower essences, homoeopathic remedies or colours may be added to augment the treatment.

and 3″ wide. On the fascia panel are from nine to twelve dials, the first is calibrated from 0 to 100 and the rest 0 to 10. Upon these dials a series of rates are placed which I will describe in a moment. On top of the box is a circular or rectangular chromed metal plate, and to one side of this is a rotating knob with a magnet attached beneath it within the box.

Once the practitioner has determined the causes of disease within the patient and the organ systems involved in each cause, he sets them out in a list for treatment. Thus he may write on the treatment card:

Staphylococcus aureus 30.44   Throat 966

This will be followed by several other pairs of rates which will be used for treatment. Each of those rates represents the frequency in radionic terms of the named factors, in this case a bacteria and a part of the body. By placing the treatment rate for staph. aureus on the first three dials of the instrument and following it with the rate for your throat, the practitioner is setting up rates or numerical values which represent in the first instance an energy pattern that will disturb the frequency of the bacteria; and the second set of numbers, representing your throat, is a directive as to where this influence should go. This also helps to strengthen the throat tissue as it is a recognition rate rather than a treatment rate. I hope you are with me so far, because the process is not at all complicated.

Having set the rates on the treatment set, the practitioner then places the patient's snippet of hair on the metal plate. He then rotates the magnet until it is in its critical rotational position. From that moment on the staph. infection which is no doubt causing a nasty sore throat, is being dispersed by the treatment rate which according to radionic theory influences the witness and thus the patient at a distance. Every so often these two sets of rates will be exchanged for others until a whole pattern of treatment has been given that deals with the causative factors that have been identified previously by radionic means.

What then in essence is a radionic treatment? Elsewhere I have defined it in this manner.

A radionic treatment is the projection of a set of coded instructions, designed to be taken up, and acted upon by the various energy fields of the patient in a way that will enable a state of harmony and health to manifest in the physical body.

The archetypal blueprint of our body is perfect, disease is a deviation from this blueprint which occurs first at the energy field level and then finally becomes physical. The vibration or frequency of the radionic rate is a way of presenting a model of the archetypal perfect pattern to the intelligence pervading the cells of the body that are presently lacking harmony, and not only reminding them of how they should function but instructing them *how* as well, thus guiding them gently towards health.

While this may be difficult to understand, and may stretch your credibility, many thousands of radionic patients throughout the world could assure you that it works. I have seen many quite remarkable cures brought about in this manner. Perhaps the most unusual of these was a Surrey housewife who had been hospitalized twice in one year for the most acute case of sinusitis I have ever seen and was due to go in again to have them 'washed out' for the third time. Her reaction to my description of radionics was not unusual, she thought it sounded far-fetched and in her mind dismissed it out of hand. Her pain mounted to even greater heights during the night, so that in desperation she contacted the practitioner I had referred her too. A witness was put in the mail, received the next morning and, unknown to the patient, she was placed on treatment immediately following the analysis, which had revealed a particularly virulent bacteria in her eustachian tubes. By lunch time the inflammation had died down; by the evening she had no sign of sinusitis. Now here was a lady who knew nothing about radionics, whose response to the idea of radionic treatment was pretty average, and who did not know she was already on treatment. She was cured in a matter of hours and had no recurrence for two years, and then only following a bad car accident abroad.

I have cited this case elsewhere in one of my other books because of its dramatic nature, let me hasten to add not all cases respond with such alacrity but it is a fact that radionic treatment can deal with disease in ways that are not open to more orthodox avenues of approach, and people can get help where other methods have failed.

Another case example further illustrates the effectiveness of radionic analysis and treatment where other approaches have failed. This patient, a male, 28 years of age, had a series of convulsions within 24 hours of being born, and difficulty in breathing. This settled down for about four months, but bouts of sickness, vomiting and mild convulsions began again when he went on to full cream milk. Over the years he showed many and varied symptoms associated with food allergies. At ten years of age he came up in large lumps which formed blisters, and was diagnosed as having chicken pox by one doctor, but this was disputed by another. His entire health history reflects this type of contradictory diagnosis. He was later classified as epileptic and placed on no fewer than four tranquilliser-type drugs, Valium and Phenobarbitone amongst them. Later a whole series of EEG scans indicated that he was not epileptic. By 1977, due to the side effects of drugs, he weighed 13½ stone, and this at a height of 5'2'' and with a light bone structure. In 1979 his mother, who fought to get to the bottom of his trouble, took him off all but the phenobarbitone and sought help from an allergist. Having identified a number of foods he was allergic to, eggs and wheat being among them, some improvements began to show and his weight dropped. The patient consulted me for a radionic analysis in February of 1984; his presenting symptoms were food allergy reactions, extreme nervousness which prevented him from venturing out, or allowing people to touch him. Any sudden or un-expected noise would cause him to drop unconscious on the spot.

His analysis showed heavy drug toxins which was not surprising, and imbalances of a marked nature in his central nervous system, gastro-intestinal tract, stomach, liver and kidneys. Radionic treatment was initiated to clear the drug toxins and to balance the various systems of the body. By March he was less jumpy and nervous, and his symptoms were abating. In June he attended a disco with no ill effects, something he could not have contemplated two months before. While his diet still has to be watched he can now venture out without the fear of collapsing and there is a vast improvement in his outlook on life.

One further case involved a health-care professional, a psychologist in fact, who led a very busy professional life, not only counselling patients but also teaching other psychologists. He suddenly became very ill, experiencing extreme lassitude and very sore throats accompanied by a strong sense of oppression and isolation. While his radionic analysis indicated a virulent infection, it was clear that he was also in a state of inner crisis and growth. My analysis of the situation fitted in with his understanding, and it was obvious from the states of his chakras and the rays that governed his subtle bodies that a shift in consciousness was taking place. By using my analysis he was able to gain a more objective view of his condition. Treatment was initiated to clear the infection and then to bring about harmony of the chakras and subtle bodies. Within a short while he was feeling greatly improved, but continued treatment for a period of one year in order to fully establish the changes that were required.

Many more cases could be cited but the above will give a general idea of how effective radionic treatment can be. If one were to ask why radionics is so effective in difficult cases, the answer would have to be because the practitioner always seeks for causes and when these are identified, treats them and not the symptoms.

7

Energy Medicines

While radionic practitioners use rates for distant healing, their repertoire is not confined solely to this method. Many make use of homoeopathic medicines derived from plants, minerals and various other substances. These remedies, which are highly diluted and prepared in such a way as to release their energy-field patterns, fit in very well with radionic treatment. Some practitioners actually prescribe remedies to be taken orally by the patient, others simply add a phial of the required remedy in the form of liquid or tablets to the rate projection, by standing it next to the patient's witness on the chrome plate. In this manner the waveform or frequency of the medicine is 'projected' or 'broadcast' to the patient along with the rates for the disease and organ system.

Back in the early years of this century, Abrams in the course of his researches found that the rate for malaria was identical to that of quinine, a drug which so successfully treats this condition. This discovery by Abrams in effect upheld the principle of homoeopathy in which 'like treats like' so you can see how radionic practitioners were attracted to homoeopathy and why many homoeopaths are sympathetic towards radionics.

In a radionic analysis there are inevitably aspects of the case in which emotional and mental factors play a part. We are psycho-somatic beings and problems are bound to arise that are psychological. Of course there are rates for these various conditions, and these are used to good effect on the

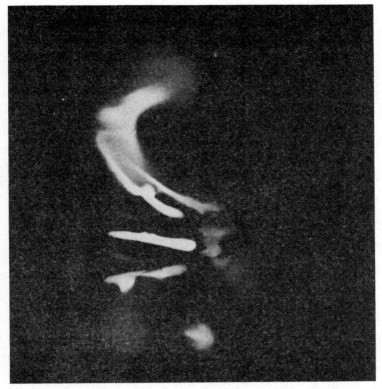

10. De La Warr radionic photograph of the Bach flower remedy, honeysuckle. This image of the flower was obtained from the radiations emitted from a bottle of the liquid remedy.

treatment sets. However most practitioners will employ the Bach flower remedies which help to heal these conditions at the inner levels where they originate, in other words the flower remedies are also energy medicines and enjoy great popularity because they can be used by lay people as well, to treat themselves or their friends and pets.

Dr. Edward Bach was a Harley Street specialist who, after many years in practice moved away from more orthodox methods and began working with flower remedies. He retired from practice in the 1930's and lived in the countryside where he began experimenting with different methods of preparing flower remedies. The flowers were picked from various plants and trees, and then prepared as medicines by two methods. Dr. Bach would either boil them in water to derive their essence or he would float the blossoms in a crystal bowl full of spring water which stood in the sun. Spirit was then added to preserve the solution which resulted from these preparations. His remedies included Mimulus, Vervain, Sweet Chestnut, Rock Rose, Water Violet, Heather and many other plants; in fact there are thirty-eight remedies altogether, one of these being Rock Water. Nobody seems to know why he decided to use this one remedy that was not derived from a plant, but in his repertory Rock Water is used for self-repression, self-denial and self-martyrdom. Essentially it is a remedy that helps to lessen inflexible states of mind.

All of the flower remedies are for emotional and mental states, and Bach arrived at his knowledge of just which flowers would have which specific effects by trying them on himself. It is reported that he was so sensitive that, if he placed the bloom of a flower on his tongue, within a short while he would experience the exact states of mind it would serve to heal. Thus he found that Mimulus was useful for fear or anxiety of a known origin, such as fear of the dark, fear of growing old or disease and death itself. Sweet Chestnut served to heal extreme mental anguish, hopelessness and despair, and Elm proved useful for feelings of inadequacy, despondency and exhaustion from over-striving for perfection. Here indeed is a remedy for those people with an overactive brow chakra.

Bach Remedies are energy medicines and as such lend themselves to use in radionic therapy. In the United States this approach has been enlarged upon to include many native species like California Poppy which is said to balance inner development, intuitive and creative abilities; and to overcome spiritual 'glamour' and over-fascination.

There are many such fine flower remedies now available thanks to Bach's pioneering work. He had rightly felt that by using the flower remedies to dispel the fears and tensions that people are subject to, the physical organism stood a far better chance of recovery. It should be obvious that these remedies treat the emotional and mental bodies, thus they balance these fields and make it easier for the physical and etheric bodies to recover.

Remedies made from gemstones are another form of energy medicine. These are prepared by placing gems in phials of alcohol for prolonged periods of time, usually in a dark container, until the vibrations or frequencies of the gem have been absorbed into the liquid. Gems have been used for healing purposes for many centuries to good effect. Ruby has been found to heal circulatory problems, anaemias, physical debility, common colds and states of collapse. Pearl is effective for gout and rheumatic conditions, asthma, menopausal trouble and inflammation. Some doctors report that it is helpful in the treatment of cataracts, a condition of the eye which almost mimics the scale of a pearl. Coral is another popular gem remedy and is used for the treatment of stomach ailments, liver disease, diabetes and nervous exhaustion.

In India where gems are commonly used in homoeopathic clinics, a colour is often ascribed to each gem remedy which does not necessarily coincide with the gem itself. This colour is used at times to guide the doctor as to which remedy or remedies he should prescribe. They check for what is known there as 'colour hunger'; that is the patient is checked through a prism or with a pendulum to see if they lack a particular colour. Then for example, if they are found to be lacking in orange and indigo, pearl and diamond remedies will be prescribed.

Colour treatment has always played an important role in radionics, and the De La Warr Laboratories produced a beautiful instrument called a Colourscope which could be used for direct or distant colour treatment. Experiments run by the laboratories over a distance of three thousand miles showed conclusively that when an individual's witness was irradiated in New York with colour, the subject in the laboratories in Oxford, who was hooked up to electronic monitoring devices, gave a clear response.

In 1878 a book appeared in America written by Dr. Edwin Babbitt, entitled *The Principles of Light and Colour*. Babbitt was a strange combination of mystic, scientist, artist and physician. He was famous in his own time for the remarkable cures he affected through colour treatments. He used blue for hepatitis, rheumatism, headaches and catarrh. Red was used for arousing the circulation of arterial blood. Yellow stimulated the nervous system, and incidentally this was the colour that George De La Warr used in his trans-Atlantic experiments. A combination of yellow and orange, according to Babbitt, proved helpful in the treatment of bronchitis, exhaustion and ulceration of the lungs.

Colour treatments are a part of every radionic practitioner's armamentarium because they readily affect the subtle bodies and chakras in a harmonious manner. Colour, like the flower remedies, is an energy medicine with a potent capacity to heal.

These then are just some of the additional factors that each radionic practitioner utilises in order to affect a cure by clearing the underlying causes of dis-ease whether they be physical or psychological.

8

Our Toxic Environment

Until very recently medicine paid little attention to toxic factors that affect people. Now there are a growing number of doctors who pay attention to human ecology and recognize the devastating effects some toxins can have on health. Radionic practitioners have always placed importance in checking each patient for toxic factors which might be undermining health, so this aspect of diagnosis is well known to them.

From time to time in the media the public is alerted to the problem of toxins. Rising amounts of lead in the atmosphere from car exhausts have prompted some governments to ban the use of lead in petrol; not unnaturally we are lagging behind here in England. Lead settles in the liver, brain, kidneys, heart, lungs, adrenals and thymus, and can cause nausea, pain, tremors, muscular weakness, headaches, insomnia, confusion and mental retardation amongst other things. If you live or work in a busy city the chances are your system will contain this toxic metal to some degree or other.

As close to home, but perhaps not so obvious, is aluminium poisoning. Cooking in aluminium ware is a guarantee that you will have this toxin in your system. The authorities are aware of this danger, and following the second World War a move was initiated to get rid of aluminium in the manufacture of cooking utensils. It did not get off the ground as vested interest was too powerful, so today the shops are full of aluminium pots and our hospitals cook food for their patients and staff in aluminium. Aspirins, deodorants and antacids all contain aluminium so it is not difficult to become contaminated. Some people seem to deal with the toxin and show no symptoms, others who are aluminium-sensitive usually have digestive problems which can become quite marked and even end up as colitis. Aluminium is a cellular, residual toxin and it causes motor nerve paralysis, constipation, skin ailments, nausea and fatty degeneration of the liver and kidneys. I have lost track of the number of patients I have found to have aluminium toxicity, and who have responded to the appropriate treatment, which includes getting stainless steel cooking ware and avoiding food cooked in aluminium. The change in their health is fast, with symptoms that have plagued them for years often disappearing in a matter of days. Another by-product of the aluminium industry is fluoride, and its toxic effects are well documented, yet it is forced upon people through the water supply as a form of medication. Fluoride, it seems, dulls the capacity to think and as a residual toxin it can cause joint pains and ultimately mottle the teeth it is supposed to harden and preserve.

Mercury-silver amalgam fillings in our teeth can prove highly toxic to some people with a sensitivity towards these substances. Mercury is well known for its toxic properties; at one time it was used in the hatting industry and the hatters used to get tremors and experience all kinds of bizarre symptoms. So marked were these symptoms that even today we use the term, 'as mad as a hatter'. Mercury waste absorbed by fish off the coast of Japan resulted in the deaths of quite a number of people and animals who ate the polluted marine life. In the United States the toxic effects of dental fillings are now being debated in the media, and research has shown that since such fillings came into use during the 1800's there has been a consistent sequential appearance of many serious and often terminal types of disease which had not been previously recorded. The metal amalgam used as a filling sets up vagrant galvanic currents in the mouth which can affect the mucous membrane of the mouth, and ions of these toxic metals are dispersed into the body by what is known as *pathological iontophoresis*. Apparently many people are not affected by these toxins; I say apparently because no one really notices the long–term effects. But people who are mercury-sensitive can literally become violently ill within hours of their first filling, in others the process is more insidious. The latter I suspect applies to more people than is realised.

Food allergies are the latest focus of interest, and it is a fact that we are in many instances sensitive to foods which have what can only be described as toxic effects upon us. These allergies often clear when the body is properly balanced and functioning at its optimum level. Two things however are worth keeping in mind, and they are tea and coffee. Both contain caffeine which is an adrenal stimulant; coffee of course has a higher content and this serves to stimulate the nervous system, the heart and the vascular system. It overloads the kidneys, particularly in older people and results in increased uric acid which causes joint pain and muscular discomfort. Tea is as a rule better tolerated, but it can cause dyspepsia and sick headaches when taken in excess. I have known individuals, particularly those who work in offices, drink up to three quarts of black coffee a day and then wonder why they are in pain from head to foot, and feeling decidedly ill most of the time. Both beverages in moderation are fine, it is the excess intake that creates problems, particularly if white sugar is added because it also stresses the body to a high degree, depleting it of vitamin B and upsetting the pancreas which can lead to other problems of a more serious nature.

Cadmium is another toxic element which is found in tea and coffee, as well as in processed meats and cigarette smoke. It can cause hypertension, enlarged heart, arteriosclerosis and kidney disease just to mention a few conditions.

This list could go on and on; most of us are aware of the toxins in our environment but I thought it worthwhile to mention these, which are so close to us in daily life that we seldom give them a thought. One of the advantages of a radionic analysis is that serious toxic states can be identified and then measures taken to clear them, whereas these toxic states may well be missed in a clinical examination. In fact few doctors would agree that aluminium, for example, can upset your health, unless of course they are practicing homoeopaths then they would be aware of that kind of problem.

As I mentioned previously, radionic practitioners have always paid attention to the possible presence of toxic factors like those listed, so they are eminently suited to deal with them effectively.

A very serious and potent source of toxins which upset people's health in a variety of ways, is from those which come from the childhood diseases. We are all familiar with the fact that rheumatic fever can leave damage in its wake in the form of a weakened heart, but how many people realise that measles, mumps, whooping cough, chicken pox and German measles can leave residual toxins that are virtually undetectable by any other means than radionics or medical radiesthesia? Very few I am sure.

I have mentioned measles toxins earlier on in the book. They can be particularly unpleasant in their effects. In the United States some 200 students died each year from a form of meningitis (brain inflammation). These were mysterious deaths in that they only seemed to affect students in their early 20's, and that no causative factor could be identified. Eventually careful investigation revealed what was termed a 'smouldering virus' which either found its way into the body by normal means or through vaccination. This so called 'smouldering virus' was measles which in some way or other became active and extremely virulent in its effect. Why, the investigators did not know, but on average it killed about 200 students a year. I think there is a clue for us in this fact alone. The toxins, as we would call the 'smouldering virus' situate themselves in the central nervous system, particularly the cerebrum, and it may well be that the intense activity of the cerebrum during college studies in some way sets up a field of energy in which these toxins become active. In other words they became energies, thus causing inflammation. Perhaps it is merely a curious coincidence, but the transpersonal self or soul is said to grasp the mental body at about 21 years of age, and this in itself causes a strong form of stimulation which combined with increased cerebral activity just tips the scales in favour of the toxin.

Mumps with its proclivity for settling in the gonads can have very disturbing effects upon the growing child, and may result in immaturity, and young men with rather high voices. Every childhood disease in fact has its toxic residues which in many instances do not seem to cause any health problems. But even if there are no disease syndromes directly attributable to these toxins they can mar a person's health for life unless they are identified and cleared with a combination of radionic and homoeopathic treatment.

There is a growing awareness of toxins in our polluted world but few would consider the dangers of amalgam mercury fillings, or aluminium pots, or toxic residues from childhood diseases because they are so close to us every day that we seldom give them a second thought. Nevertheless they constitute a real hazard to health.

9

How Does Radionics Work?

This question is still being debated despite the fact that radionics in its present form has been practised for many decades now throughout the world, and quite a number of people have theorised as to how radionics works. It is safe to say that radionics is directly related to thought, thus there is a mental component active in both the diagnostic and therapeutic aspects of radionics. It also involves field theories drawn in part from science and in part from the more esoteric areas of religion and philosophy.

I have already touched upon field theory very briefly earlier on in the book, and I do not think there is anything to be gained by expanding on this to any degree. We have seen that fields generate objects and life-forms, and that each life-form has its own field. The life or L-Fields of one person can, by thought, affect another person or object at a distance. No one is sure how this works but it is accepted generally that human consciousness can influence the strength of other biogravitational fields over distances great or small. Perhaps you have deliberately stared at the back of a person's head to make them turn around and look at you, or you have responded to the impulse to turn and look behind you, only to find someone is staring at you. This is something we have all experienced and it is a field-phenomenon that involves the use of mind and thought. The Australian Aborigine who lives in a vast world that is filled with silence for the most part, has this ability developed to a very high degree, so much so that if he has trained himself in the art, he can use it to literally read the mind of another individual, or to heal them from a distance. Similarly he can 'see' game animals a long way off, despite the fact that they are not visible to physical sight. These abilities are common to many tribal societies, or used to be. Our so called civilisation seems to dull and atrophy the subtle sense mechanisms needed for this form of perception. But it can be developed with the proper training, and utilised in distant diagnosis and to heal.

Today, if we are to look for a clearer explanation of the radionic phenomena and to understand just how diagnosis and treatment can be carried out from a distance, and how radionic photographs showing cross-sections of human tissues, taken over thousands of miles from the subject, come into being, we are going to have to look to quantum physics. This of course is enough to immediately deter most people from seeking any further for an explanation, but curiously enough modern physics seems to echo many of the ideas found in the ancient Mystery Teachings. Quantum theory states that *you cannot move without influencing everything in your universe.* We might note that the Bible says "not a sparrow falls without it being noticed." Quantum theory then goes on to say that, *you cannot even observe anything without changing the object and even yourself.*

When a radionic practitioner places your witness in his instrument and tunes in to you, an effect has already taken place. As quantums of energy flow from the practitioner to you, modified by the instrument with its rate settings, then that energy causes the atoms of your body to vibrate thus changing your field and ultimately the dis-eased particles. If this is done properly then your health will be restored. The ancients said that we are one, we are all connected; modern physics speaks of quantum interconnectedness, it is one and the same thing and this is what is utilised in radionics.

As I said before, we think so much in physical terms because we live in a physical universe, and it is obvious to us that space separates one person from another. However at the higher levels of consciousness, there is no time or space as we experience them in the physical world. So when a practitioner tunes into you, the patient, there is an immediate proximity at the level of the mind where the work is carried out. The mind of the practitioner has access to otherwise hidden data regarding your health which he uses to your advantage in order to restore health.

By now you may be wondering if such techniques could be misused. The answer to that has to be yes, they can! But it is a curious fact that anyone who misuses this ability frequently finds themselves in trouble of one kind or another, and often the skill to diagnose and treat effectively at a distance disappears. Sensitivity of this kind has to be treated as a gift to be used in the service of humanity, anything less constitutes misuse.

I will say no more about how radionics works; it is a complex subject and one that I have gone into in some detail in my various books on the subject. For the reader who wishes to pursue this avenue of investigation further those books may prove helpful, and I would suggest that a paperback entitled *Space-Time and Beyond* by Bob Toben makes delightful and amusing reading because it illustrates quantum physics with large format cartoons and a minimum of text. In other words it is a painless way of coming to a better understanding of the principles that lie behind action at a distance and radionic healing techniques.

10

Body – Mind – Spirit

We will return now to that component of the analysis chart that I left uninterpreted earlier on. If you look at it you will see a series of four circles surmounted by a triangle. Each of the three smaller circles surrounded by the ovoid represents one of the bodies or vehicles that we as humans utilise in what the sages of the East call the three worlds. The lower circle represents the physical and etheric bodies as a unit. The next circle represents the emotional body and the one above that the mental. The larger circle above the ovoid is the transpersonal self and the triangle represents the spirit within. The ovoid itself symbolises the personality or the sum total of energies of the lower-self consisting of the mental, emotional, etheric and physical bodies.

This is a construct of the esoteric constitution of man which can be found in many spiritual teachings, and it is a model which can be used to good effect in coming to understand the way people function. Above all it shows the quality of energy present in each body, and these energies create our character and to a great extent determine the way we approach and handle life. The way in which the various energy fields interact of course is a prime source of physical and psychological disease, so this aspect of the radionic analysis can be of considerable import to the individual who has a background in the esoteric teachings and is not only prepared but *capable* of cooperating with the practitioner on the inner levels in order to restore harmony and health. This presupposes a great deal of knowledge on the part of the practitioner, and no small amount on the part of the patient. This makes it a peculiarly specialised aspect of radionics at this time, but it is one which will, at some future date, prove to be of remarkable import. It is this which can make radionics a truly holistic approach to healing, in that it does literally deal with the whole man.

We have considered the analysis of the physical–etheric organ systems of the body and the states of the chakras and how they influence health, and the subtle bodies. Now by looking at the energy pattern of each body we can get a deeper picture altogether. In my interpretation of these energies in our hypothetical case I am not going to go into a lot of detail. Suffice to say that there are five volumes on this subject alone written by Alice A. Bailey and published by Lucis Press.

In her books the energies that qualify each body are known as rays, of which there are seven. They crop up again and again in various religions — in the Bible for example they are called the seven spirits before the throne of God. Jacob Boehme the Christian mystic referred to them as the seven fountain spirits. We should just think of them as seven qualities of energy which give rise to seven basic characters of man. Each energy is numbered one to seven, and I am going to say no more about them at this point except that the energies 2, 4 and 6 tend to work harmoniously together but can conflict with energies 1, 3, 5 and 7 which also work well together. Each ray or energy has its virtuous qualities, its vices and its glamours, which are its deceptive qualities. As I said previously I do not intend to list all of these; if you are interested sufficiently you can read the available literature on the subject. However as I interpret John Doe's rays you will get an idea of the nature of some of these energies and how they mould our lives. So let us see what these energies tell us about this individual.

He has a 2nd ray transpersonal self which would incline him towards teaching or work in a healing profession. He would be intuitive, patient and concerned with truth, but there would be, at times, indifference to others and he may be contemptuous of their shortcoming especially in the mental sphere. The 2nd ray frequently lays him open to fears of all kinds, and leaves him with a sense of inadequacy and inferiority. He suffers from all kinds of anxiety and is never really satisfied with his level of attainment. In certain situations John Doe can adopt a self-effacing posture, and with his tact might well make a fine ambassador.

With his 5th ray mind he will look for accurate statements about things. He will tend towards being independent, upright and will have plenty of common sense. At times he may lack sympathy and hold narrow views with a certain arrogance. As a rule he will be punctual, but if you are late or cross his path he will have difficulty in forgiving you. The 5th ray tends to confer a rather critical nature, and he is the kind of man who wants proof of statements made by others.

His emotional body is on the 6th ray and this often causes him to be rather idealistic and devotional, and if his 5th ray mind does not hold sway he might well make hasty decisions and come to rapid conclusions that he later regrets. He has a marked reluctance to make changes and tends to be rather fixed in his opinions. Inevitably there is too much intensity of feeling and this is one of the problems that causes his solar plexus chakra to be so overactive. Rigid attitudes can lead to a rigid body, so arthritic conditions may appear if more flexible approaches to life situations are not adopted.

John Doe's physical–etheric body is on the 3rd ray. This confers on him sincerity, a clear intellectual capacity and as a rule it makes philosophic studies easy. However he is a person who may see so many angles to a question that it paralyses all action. With the 5th ray mind he is going to be critical of others and even himself at times, and this is heightened by the 3rd ray physical. He will always be a very busy person and may well talk and move rapidly, and may be preoccupied with material matters and making money which is the forte of 3rd ray people. Frequently it places them squarely in the business world.

Finally he has a 4th ray personality; now this means that he has a capacity to bring harmony to conflicting situations (a plus for any ambassador) and because of this ray may find that both his personal and business life throw up conflicts so that he has to deal with them. He will have a good sense of colour and proportion and an innate capacity to know when things are correctly balanced or not. The 4th ray confers changeableness, vagueness and impracticality; it can diffuse interests to the point where John Doe's energies are scattered through too many projects, especially as his 3rd ray physical makes him a 'busy body' anyhow. One thing for sure, he will always be at war within. In constant combat as the forces of inertia and activity sway back and forth creating what amounts at times to great nervous stress and psychological tension. His conversations may well vary from brilliant discourses to gloomy silences.

Even from this brief outline it is clear that a great deal of information can be derived from knowing which rays or energies qualify each body. Every ray predisposes us to certain strengths and weaknesses and constitutes principles of limitation, as well as endowing us with certain gifts and capacities. Just how we use these various energies is up to us, but in their misuses we find those vibrations which will activate the seeds of dis-ease within us. As I have previously stated this is a very brief outline of the rays, it would be quite possible to write many pages tracing all of the interactions and blockages in the ray makeup of John Doe, and delineating their relationship to the chakras and the state of his physical health. This would only be done however if he were able to profit from the information by taking an active part in his own health care.

It should be clear by now that radionics is a truly holistic healing art, and one thing is certain — we shall see the increasing use of this approach to health in the years to come as patients demand to know what lies at the root of their health problems.

Publishers note: Radionic analysis of the rays was introduced into radionics by the author with the publication of *Radionics: Science or Magic*? He has made a 23 year study of this complex subject, and to our knowledge is the only radionic practitioner who is qualified to enter into this type of detail with any accuracy. It is not therefore a part of every radionic practitioner's approach.

An Overview

Despite the fact that radionics in its original form as the Electronic Reaction of Abrams, was one of the most revolutionary breakthroughs to occur in medicine during the early part of this century, it has not enjoyed full recognition. Perhaps it was an idea too far ahead of its time, and quite possibly the calibre of practitioner required for this work faded out of the picture as medicine in particular became more and more deeply embedded and bogged down in a physical approach to health problems and their subsequent cure. The prophecy of an age of miracle drugs has not been fulfilled, rather the opposite. The increase of iatrogenic (doctor caused) disease is now epidemic and people, quite naturally, are looking elsewhere for relief. By conservative estimates ten per cent of all people in hospital are there as a result of the harmful effects of prescribed drugs; other sources put the figure as high as twenty-five per cent.

The recent and rapidly growing interest in alternative healing methods is a sign of change, that will in itself force orthodoxy to reconsider its position, its beliefs and above all its approach to healing. Predictably it will at first attempt to procure the various alternative methods, and lay claim to them. We witnessed this recently, when statements by the Prince of Wales about the 'dinosaur' of modern medicine forced the British Medical Association into making defensive noises on television and elsewhere in the media, regarding their attitude to alternative methods of healing. They have been forced to say they will look into them, that they appear to have merit; but if you want alternative forms of treatment they urge you to go to a medical doctor, which is quite a contradictory statement in itself. In the 1960's they admitted in the media that they knew nothing much about treating back problems, but they were hard at work researching the matter. In the meantime, until they had come up with some results they advised the public to keep away from osteopaths and chiropractors. I wonder how this form of mentality is going to cope with New Age approaches to healing, or if indeed it can in its present posture of superiority.

Whatever modern medicine and medical politics may think, we are entering an era in which the holistic approach is being demanded by a rapidly increasing number of people. Witness for example the growing popularity of homoeopathy with its use of remedies that seek to heal the body instead of to suppress symptoms. Radionics like homoeopathy looks at the whole man, not just a fragment of him.

Elsewhere I have written that radionics is an entelechtic approach to healing. What does that mean? Well, 'entelechy' is defined in the medical dictionary as 'Completion; full development or realization; the complete expression of some function. A *vital principle operating in living creatures as a directive spirit*'. Radionics, by its very nature, is an entelechtic approach to healing. It is concerned with the whole man, it looks at him in both physical and paraphysical terms, it recognizes man's spiritual nature. It pays direct attention to the unitary force within the structures of man and treats this force with measures that are gentle and non-invasive. Above all it deals with the causative factors of ill health which are more often than not unidentifiable by any other means.

Abrams, the father of radionics, discovered the principles of Electronic Medicine. He established through his researches that diseases were vibratory energy states, and could be treated with energy, whether in the form of homoeopathic medicines or by electromagnetic means. This is a far cry from the cellular theory of disease which in the light of modern physics is quite outmoded. Yet orthodox medicine clings to this view, backed to the hilt of course by the drug companies.

Radionics has always seen disease conditions in terms of energy, and now that we also see man in a similar light, there is no doubt that radionics will have a vital role to play during the coming decades as people and health care professionals alike become aware of this.

Suggested Reading

New Worlds Beyond the Atom by Langston Day & George De La Warr (Vincent Stuart Ltd).

Matter in the Making by Langston Day & George De La Warr (Vincent Stuart Ltd).

Radionics and the Subtle Anatomy of Man by David V. Tansley, D.C.

Radionics — Interface with the Ether Fields by David V. Tansley, D.C.

Dimensions of Radionics by David V. Tansley, D.C.

Radionics: Science or Magic? by David V. Tansley, D.C.

Chakras — Rays and Radionics by David V. Tansley, D.C.

(These five titles published by C.W. Daniels Co. Ltd.)

The Chain of Life by Dr. Guyon Richards (C.W. Daniels Co. Ltd).

An Introduction to Medical Radiesthesia and Radionics by Vernon Wethered (C.W. Daniels Co. Ltd).

Report on Radionics by Edward Russell (Neville Spearman Ltd).

Healing through Radionics by L. Dower & E. Baerlein (Thorsons Ltd).

The Raiment of Light by David V. Tansley, D.C. (Routledge & Kegan Paul).

Space-Time and Beyond by Bob Toben (E.P. Dutton. New York).

Mysticism and the New Physics by Michael Talbot (Routledge & Kegan Paul).

Planet Medicine by Richard Grossinger (Shambhala).

Space, Time & Medicine by Larry Dassey, M. D. (Shambhala).

The Pattern of Health by Aubrey Westlake (to be reprinted by Element Books 1985).

Principles & Practice of Radiesthesia by Abbé Mermet (Watkins).

Contact Addresses

The De La Warr Laboratories
Raleigh Park Road
Oxford
Oxon

Advanced Radionic Consultants
David V. Tansley DC
38 South Street
Chichester
Sussex

The Radionic Association
Baerlein House
Goose Green
Deddington
Oxford
OX5 4SZ